ENZYMES

The Fountain of Life

For more specific information please contact:

USA

Naturally Vitamin Supplements
Phone   1-800-899-4499
Fax   1-602-991-0551
Internet   http://www.naturallyvitamins.com

Mike Williams, M.D.
H-822 Monticello Place
Evanston, IL 60201

D. A. Lopez, M.D.
Phone   1-619-454-3642
Fax   1-619-454-8723
CompuServe   74344,461

Germany

MUCOS Pharma, Germany
Phone   +49-8171-518-0
Fax   +49-8171-52008
CompuServe   100060,1177
Internet   http://www.mucos.de

Medical Enzyme Research Foundation, Germany
Phone   +49-8171-518-300
Fax   +49-8171-518-303

ENZYMES

The Fountain of Life

D.A. Lopez, M.D.

R.M. Williams, M.D. Ph.D.

K. Miehlke, M.D.

The Neville Press, Inc.

1994

ENZYMES
The Fountain of Life

FIRST ENGLISH EDITION

Type Setting: Ing. Büro Söllner GmbH, D 81369 München
Printed by: Weber Offset GmbH, D 80993 München

Printed in Germany

ISBN 1-884303-00-5
3 4 5 6 7 8 9   EZ/NP   99 98 97 96

D. A. Lopez, M.D.

Associate Clinical Professor of Medicine at UCSD Medical School, San Diego, California

Director, Regional Hansens Disease Center, San Diego, California

Dr. Lopez is a practicing physican in San Diego, California. He completed his residency training at the U.S. Naval Hospital in San Diego and his fellowship training at the Armed Forces Institute of Pathology in Washington, DC. Dr. Lopez also completed additional graduate training in tropical medicine at the Gorgas Memorial Institute in Panama. He is a former U.S. Navy medical corps Captain and currently an Associate Clinical Professor of medicine at UCSD, with many years of experience teaching medical students and residents. He has published various medical and scientific articles and lectured extensively across the U.S and overseas. He is also the Director of the Regional Hansens Disease Center in San Diego, CA.

During his entire medical career, Dr. Lopez has had a particular interest in the natural immune defenses of the human body, the immunology of infectious diseases and the immunology of cancer. He has continuously participated in immunologic research during the past 18 years.

Dr. Lopez has extensively studied the biologic response modifiers and their uses in medicine, particularly their effects in the treatment of some types of cancer and of immune disorders.

During the past five years, he has been involved in a comprehensive study of the emerging field of *immunoenzymology*. In this book he joins other highly experienced physicians in the review and analysis of the world's medical literature on this field and together they bring their findings to the American public.

R. Michael Williams, M.D., Ph.D.

Professor of Medicine, Northwestern University Medical School
Chairman, Board of Scientific Counselors
Cancer Treatment Research Foundation
Senior Medical Director and Chief Medical Officer
Cancer Treatment Centers of America

Dr. R. Michael Williams has been studying enzymes since high school. The launching of Sputnik led to a program to involve students in research at medical schools. Williams was selected to measure urokinase activity on artificial blood clots. During college at Yale University, he wrote his honors thesis on antibodies to acetylcholinesterase and published this work in the *Proceedings of the National Academy of Sciences*. He received a masters degree at Yale where he studied thymus derived cells. In medical school at Harvard University, he studied the genetic control of immune responses and cancer. As the first graduate student of the Nobel Laureate professor Baruj Benacerraf, Dr. Williams received his Ph.D degree in immunology from Harvard in 1974. He then trained in hematology and medical oncology, worked at the Peter Bent Brigham Hospital and the Dana Farber Cancer Institute, and was an Assistant Professor of Medicine at Harvard Medical School.

Dr. Williams later became a Professor of Medicine and Chief of Medical Oncology at Northwestern University Medical School in Chicago. In 1989 he was a co-founder of the Cancer Treatment Center of America and continues as its Senior Medical Director and Chief Medical Officer. Now he considers his most important task to be that of Founding Director and Chairman of the Board of Scientific Counselors of the Cancer Treatment Research Foundation. This nonprofit research foundation is dedicated to conducting and supporting rigorous scientific study of cancer therapies based on immunology, molecular genetics and nutrition. A major goal of the CTRF is to expedite the translation of this basic research to benefit cancer patients. Examples of initiatives supported by the CTRF are the Nutrition Oncology Adjuvant Treatment study group and the annual Adjuvant Nutrition in Cancer Treatment Symposium.

Klaus Miehlke, M.D.

Professor of Rheumatology
Board of the German Society for Internal Medicine
Scientific Advisory Council of the State Medical Board of Registration in Germany
Registration Board of the German Federal Ministry of Health
Member of the New York Academy of Sciences

Dr. Miehlke is a Professor of Rheumatology and author of 180 medical publications. He was the Medical Director and Senior Physician of the Rheumatological Clinic in Wiesbaden, Germany from 1961 to 1988.

He obtained his clinical training at the University Medical Centers in Gottingen and in Nuremberg, Germany, in Zurich, Switzerland and at the University of Pennsylvania in Philadelphia. After obtaining his post-doctoral lecturing qualifications for Internal Medicine at the University of Mainz in Mainz, Germany, he was appointed as an Extraordinary Professor in 1974.

Dr. Miehlke is a very experienced internist and rheumatologist with a distinguished academic career and superb clinical credits. He has delivered over 800 scientific lectures in Germany and elsewhere.

Dr. Miehlke is an internationally recognized expert in systemic enzyme therapy with many years of clinical experience in the use of oral hydrolytic enzymes for the treatment of various acute and chronic rheumatologic conditions.

In addition to his distinguished clinical and academic career, Dr. Miehlke has an appointment as a Standing Member of the Board of the German Society for Internal Medicine (Resident Protocolist), is a member of the Registration Committee of the German Federal Mininstry of Health and a long standing member of the Scientific Advisory Council of the State Medical Board of Registration in Germany. He is also a member of the New York Academy of Sciences.

Acknowledgments

This book deals with the unique relationship between the medical disciplines of immunology and enzymology. As such, it represents the first comprehensive book on the emerging field of *immunoenzymology*. Our work would not have been possible without the prior work and publications of thousand of scientists and authors before us. We wish to thank the many investigators who conducted the original clinical and laboratory research dealing with the various aspects of immunoenzymology and systemic enzyme therapy over a period of many years.

We owe a special debt of gratitude to those who helped in the preparation of this manuscript and who offered their expertise, constructive criticism and advice, and those who kindly shared substantial portions of their personal collections and reviews.

We offer special thanks to those friends in the United States and in Europe who helped us with the manuscript and the literature search.

Our sincere thanks to Dr. O. Pecher for his invaluable help, Dr. Ed W. Beese for the translations from the German, and to Dr. Raul Ahumada for his review of the manuscript, constructive criticism and translations from the German and Italian. We also wish to thank Dr. Frank Gareis for his corrections and kind suggestions.

Many other friends and associates helped us one way or another with the manuscript and we ask their forgiveness for not being able to name them all.

Finally, we wish to thank our families for their understanding and support during the many hours of work required for this publication.

Contents

Figures and Tables Index

Introduction

Why enzymes?

Enzymes are fascinating from a medical, scientific and even philosophical point of view. Enzyme systems constitute an essential component of life for humans, animals, plants and all microorganisms. They can only be formed from organic living matter. Enzymes are required for the proper and normal functioning of every organ system. They direct, accelerate, modify or retard all body functions. They do so in a unique, step-by-step, highly efficient, safe and remarkably economical manner. This step-by-step function insures safety, efficiency, and in terms of energy expenditure, economy.

Enzymes serve as the body's labor force to perform every single function required for our daily activities and are required to keep us alive. They are responsible for all of the functions of every organ system in our bodies. At the same time, they are most important in supporting our body defenses and immune system to protect us from harmful forces and specific dangers to our health. The immune system depends heavily on enzymes to conduct its protective functions. For example, in the complement system, one of the most important 'defense/attack' branches of the immune system that will be discussed later in the book, there are nine step-by-step primary components involving 27 known subproteins, 22 of which are enzymes! (Figure 1)

In addition to our immune and defense systems, we require enzymes not only to eat, digest and absorb our nutrients, but also to see, hear, smell, taste, breathe and move. Enzymes are required for our blood and coagulation system, cardiovascular functions, kidneys, liver, elimination of toxic products, excretion, reproduction, etc. They are required even to think, dream or for sexual excitement or activity! When enzyme activity stops, life stops and the person or organism dies!

It is obvious that medical science should have as much knowledge as possible regarding a body system so important to our health, to our lives and to our body's ability to protect us from illnesses. By measuring enzymes present in our blood and other tissues, physicians can learn how the body is functioning, alert us about illness and monitor response to the various treatments. A healthy enzyme system is also important in disease prevention. Physicians are continuously learning to better evaluate how our bodies are functioning, which enzymes are involved in the various functions, and which abnormal enzyme mechanisms in our bodies result in diseases. They are also beginning to learn how to manipulate enzymes at the most basic tissue or cellular levels where they may be defective and cause disease. Likewise, they are learning how to administer enzymes to correct or even prevent these disease causing abnormalities.

For the moment, let us concentrate on a more important issue. What are enzymes? Why are they important to us? How do they help us?

What are enzymes?

Living cells and tissues require basic nutrients and essential substances to divide, grow and perform their normal activities. Most of these substances are synthesized from components of ingested food, water and other nutritional supplements, or from breakdown products of tissues. The biochemical reactions to synthesize the basic elements required by living cells depend on a steady supply of energy from these sources. Ordinarily, this energy is supplied by a step-by-step oxidation of food components. In addition, the biochemical reactions themselves sometimes release energy. During times of stress or disease, there is an increased demand for the nutrients and essential supplies required by cells.

Without very special helpers and at normal body temperature, it would be impossible for the cells and tissues to perform all the essential biochemical reactions required fast enough to meet the basic needs of the body. Fortunately, very specific and remarkable helpers initiate, accelerate and terminate these biochemical reactions. The helpers are highly specific organic substances which have evolved in living organisms and developed the capacity of perfoming these accelerating tasks to perfection via remarkable and specific catalytic actions. These remarkable substances are called *enzymes.*

Enzymes are catalysts. They make things work faster. For example, the chemistry of the body is all about utilizing one substance to produce another. Let us call it turning chemical A into chemical B. The biochemical reaction to do this may require energy or release energy, depending on whether molecules A or B contain their own energy.

Regardless of whether energy is required or released, the reaction time is shortened by its specific enzyme, without the enzyme itself being used up. The reaction is accelerated through the use of enzymes. For example, an enzyme can help a reaction that converts substance A to substance B and vice versa:

A + enzyme + energy ----> B + unchanged enzyme

or

B + enzyme ----> A+ energy + unchanged enzyme

This acceleration without consumption is the nature of a catalyst. For practical purposes, most biochemical reactions require enzymes since the reaction from A ----> B might take hundreds of years without them.

Why are enzymes important to us?

To an amazingly large extent, enzymes are responsible for our health! Biochemists have described them as 'the body's labor force' or 'the life energy' of all organisms. And yet, medicine has paid only limited attention to these vital components of our bodies. When enzymes were studied in medical school by the authors, the emphasis was placed on their function as digestive elements from the pancreas and gastrointestinal tract, and on their role in diagnosis. We were taught in medical school that oral enzymes were indicated only for digestive problems and that they were not indicated for any other medical conditions 'because they were not absorbed'. Unfortunately, in the United States and other countries, this was generally accepted as 'medical dogma' and the potential and importance of all enzymes for actual medical treatment was nearly overlooked for decades.

During the past several years there has been a resurgence of interest on enzymes for medical diagnosis and treatment, as well as for other uses, based on the development of new technology. These technological breakthroughs have led to remarkable advances. Medicine has again, in full force, entered the field of therapeutic enzymes. However, in the United States, it appears that there has been less interest in the use of therapeutic medical enzymes than in Japan and Europe. On the other hand, in the United States there has been phenomenal progress in the use of enzymes for medical diagnosis, and in industry, in contrast to their use for medical treatment.

During the past decade, enzyme usage in diagnostic tests has increased dramatically in medical practice worldwide. Even more important, new and highly promising clinical indications for systemic enzyme treatment are being reported. In addition to their use for digestive disorders in the United States and other countries, enzymes are now widely used in the treatment of various types of blood clots, particularly those causing heart attacks and occlusions of the veins of the legs, and in the treatment of several congenital deficiency diseases. Enzyme use for specific subtypes of emphysema, a respiratory disorder, was recently approved. A number of other diseases have been found to be caused by abnormalities, defects or deficiencies of specific enzyme systems. Knowledge in this field has nearly exploded with the help of newer technology, such as the genetic engineering techniques involving recombinant DNA. The importance of enzymes in such deficiency diseases was eloquently emphasized in the movie "Lorenzo's Oil", dealing with progressive neurological changes and suffering of a patient and his family resulting from a defect in an enzyme system.

This book will review the subject of enzymes in simple terms which may be understood by the lay public as well as by interested professionals in the medical, paramedical and scientific fields. It represents a comprehensive review of the scientific world literature dealing with the subject of enzymes. The book starts with a philosophical discussion of the importance of enzymes to life. It then moves through the history of enzymes and reviews advances in enzymology. Current worldwide uses in diagnosis, treatment and prevention of diseases are also discussed. Emphasis is placed on the importance of enzymes to our health as applicable to our metabolism and internal functions. Considerable time is spent reviewing the role of enzymes in our body defenses, particularly their role in the immune system and in inflammation. We will touch on the basic nature and function of enzymes, making a careful attempt to explain and simplify basic biochemical and medical concepts and terms.

Medical uses of enzymes in other countries will be reviewed, including various forms of systemic enzyme treatments. Experiences and conclusions from clinical studies and clinical use in those countries will be reviewed in detail. Much can be learned from these other countries regarding treatments of difficult illnesses and of conditions where modern medicine does not offer particularly good treatments at present.

The book also discusses basic aspects about nutrition as related to enzymes. Nutrition alone should not be construed as a substitute to good and proper medical care. However, proper nutrition plays a very important role in health and is an essential component of any form of treatment, particularly for advanced or debilitating illnesses. The authors review specific concepts regarding proper nutrition which will support the importance of enzymes in the diet, particularly if fresh and unprocessed foods are consumed whenever possible. Fresh, natural, unprocessed foods will supply us with necessary enzymatic products and will provide the essential enzyme helpers known as coenzymes (vitamins, trace elements and minerals) required by our bodies to function properly.

Overview of enzymes in health and disease

Most people are born with a properly functioning enzyme system which, in turn, helps perform all of the tasks of the body, from the simplest to the most complex and important. So far, only around 3,000 enzymes are known in the human body, but many thousands more which have not yet been discovered are felt to be responsible for keeping us alive. Their importance is enormous. They represent our life energy! What is their origin? How far can we go to trace this enzymatic life force activity for a single person? This book reviews the role of enzymes in the origin of life and their specialization through evolution.

To illustrate some of the many functions of enzymes in our lives, we will start with one example. For our purposes we will look briefly at a process that is a favorite of all humans. The subject is love. Enzymes are present in the pheromones that produce attraction, sexual excitement and arousal between man and woman. Numerous enzymes contribute to the marvel of sexuality, and to the wonder of sex. Enzymes provide the energy source for the sperm to travel to the ovum and, upon contact, another enzyme opens a 'door' for the sperm to penetrate, while yet another one seals the opening to prevent other spermatozoa from entering. Fertilization and conception require a highly coordinated sequence of enzymatic activity, like a team of enzymes playing in harmony to join the genetic material of the father and mother, and progress to the formation of the embryo. Thus, human life begins with the remarkable magic of enzymes creating a most beautiful and wonderful artistic performance that leads to the baby. Within the nucleus of each cell, the baby has 23 chromosomes from the father and 23 from the mother. The hereditary blueprint from the parents is coded in each chromosome and will determine a final and unique expression in this child, representing a blend of all of the family traits. The genes passed from the parents and present along the chromosomes determine the actual coding. The DNA molecules within the chromosomes constitute the actual memory of the cell. Within a single cell there are roughly 100,000 genes, the majority of which code for enzymes. Each gene, whether structural, receptor, etc., is associated with an enzyme action, and is predetermined to perform a specific function. With the help of enzymes, numerous cells reproduce by division every second to form new cells with exactly the same genetic composition. These will replace older ones. At the same time, many older cells are dying. All of the required labor for the renewal and elimination is performed by enzymes encoded in those genes. Although a limited number of other cells do not actually divide to form new ones, such as some brain cells and the ova within the ovaries, they are maintained in a state of good health by our enzymes.

Within the sum total of our bodies, enzymes work constantly like a majestic orchestra conducting a splendid symphony in perfect harmony. This perfect equilibrium keeps us active and preserves our health, performing all functions through a delicate and yet phenomenal system of checks and balances. They help to build new cells and new tissues as needed, and to remove waste as required. They also are the key elements of our immune systems and body surveillance network. Together with the immune cells and mediators, they help to destroy harmful elements, such as

Overview of complement cascade sequence and actions (Each component has various subunits not listed)

Response to immune complex	Types of actions after activation	C'3 Actions	C'5 - C'6 Actions	C'7 Actions	C'8 - C'9 Actions
Complement fixation and activation	**Regulated** ⇒ ⇒ G O O D	Coating of organisms Neutrophil chemotaxis Immune adherence Phagocytosis	Normal histamine release Increased vascular permeability Release of cells and humoral elements to site of inflammation	Increased neutrophil chemotaxis Re-enforce phagocytosis Stabilization and preparation of complement for **cell or germ destruction (lysis)**	**Enzyme release** ⇒ **Destruction of bacteria, viruses, parasites, fungi and cancer cells by lysis.** ⇒ Additional histamine release ⇒ Feed back to stop further destruction of normal tissue by complement
+ C'1 + C'4 + C'2	→ Activation →	+ C'3	+ C'5 + C'6	+ C'7	+ C'8 - C'9
Complement binding sites exposed and first component's enzymatic activity is converted to active form thus releasing the cascade	**Unregulated** ⇒ ⇒ B A D	Excessive anaphylotoxin generation Vasodilatation Cell degranulation Release of mediators Leukocyte thrombi	Abnormal histamine release Excessive release of cells and humoral elements to site of inflammation Shock	Blood vessel clogging with excessive cellular elements	**Destruction of normal cells by lysis** (Example: hemolytic anemia) Destruction of transplant cells

⇒ **Lysis**

Immune ▶

Complex ◀

Figure 1: Pathway of the complement cascade with emphasis on its normal functions and unregulated consequences infections, pollution, carcinogens, and other noxious agents that develop within our bodies, either as a result of our own metabolism, or from exposure, ingestion, inhalation, administration, etc. They eliminate early cancerous cells developing in the body. They are essential for repairing damaged tissues, controlling excessive inflammation, inducing proper fluidity in our blood which prevents abnormal coagulation, and many more functions. They perform their functions as biocatalysts that are not used up in their labor, but are able to break down the substrates required by the body (nutrients, trace elements, body proteins, damaged tissues, etc.), and then use and reuse the breakdown components as building blocks for all our needs. The enzymes work as tireless, highly-skilled workers on a conveyor belt, dismantling, controlling, protecting, destroying, eliminating, reassembling or performing whatever we need in order to exist day and night. After completing their missions and life-spans, enzymes themselves age and are constantly dismantled by other enzymes and then replaced in our bodies. In good health, there is always a new supply of enzymes able and ready to keep on working.

The many complex major pathways, such as coagulation, immunity, neuroendocrine system, etc., which the body utilizes for all our needs, also function via the body's labor force of enzymes. In an automobile assembly line, when a worker fails and the chain is interrupted, the final product suffers. Likewise, it is also easy to see how and why a mistake in an enzyme can affect a particular step-by-step system to which that enzyme belongs, and lead to errors which can cause disease. It is also easy to see the tremendous importance of enzymes in the general scheme of our health and the health of all living organisms.

The enzyme systems, our organs, tissues and nutrition are interdependent. We also depend to a significant extent on our nutrition to obtain essential factors that are required by the enzymes to function properly. These are the coenzymes already mentioned. Fortunately, we can get some of our enzymes in our food. Unfortunately, the heat of stove or microwave cooking, high refining of foodstuffs and pasteurization will kill the enzymes in foods! Many other harmful activities we perform, such as smoking, exposure to carcinogens, excessive exposure to sunlight, use of dangerous drugs, exposure to toxic substances, radiation, and possibly other agents, will damage some of our internal enzymes. When the food enzymes are not sufficient, our digestive glands have to work extra hard to make up the difference and complete the digestion. If we do not help by eating properly, the digestive glands, and sometimes the thyroid, work extra hard day after day and eventually become enlarged and less efficient. They then utilize more and more of the basic elements (amino acid chains and coenzymes) taking them away from the other organs and tissues of the body which also require them for their own metabolic enzymatic activity to function properly. This results in a shortfall of basic supplies on both sides. Some scientists feel this shortfall in metabolic enzymes contributes to some of our modern society diseases, such as degenerative disorders (osteoarthritis, emphysema, osteoporosis, gastrointestinal disorders, Alzheimer's, etc.) and to some autoaggressive diseases (collagen vascular diseases such as rheumatoid arthritis, lupus, scleroderma, etc.), and to cancer. Whether this is the case or not remains to be proven by science. It is highly logical, however, that alterations, defects, absence, insufficiency or excesses in enzymes contribute one way or another to all diseases.

Enzymes as biological response modifiers

During the past few years, medicine has entered a new era in therapy. The emphasis has been placed in treatment with substances which stimulate, replace or duplicate the actions of the internal cellular mediators which our bodies use in conjunction with our immune systems to protect us from harm. They are substances of biological origin administered to patients or to a biological system in order to improve or modify a natural body system response, generally of the immune function. These agents are collectively called Biological Response Modifiers or BRM's. These biological treatments are increasingly considered as safe, natural and rational approaches that stimulate our normal biological responses and defenses. They are purported simply to help an immune system that has been sluggish or overtaxed by providing these new immune stimulants or mediator agents to aid in the fight. The BRM's are actually similar to immune mediators in our bodies, or are capable of boosting our normal immune functions. Thus, it is thought that they allow the rest of the body defenses to reconstitute themselves and take over. The introduction of BRM's to modern medicine represents a tremendous advance in treatment and it can be expected that their use will increase more and more as we discover ways in which our defenses function. Results of their use appear most encouraging. These substances work together with our internal natural body enzymes as immune system stimulants. Therapeutic enzymes themselves also are considered to be important Biological Response Modifiers.

BRM's have been used in clinical trials in a number of (autoimmune) conditions, cancer and HIV disease. Most of them are of plant, microbial and, to a lesser extent, animal origin. In addition to therapeutic enzymes, another important group of BRM's consists of substances called *colony stimulating factors*. These are being extensively studied at present and used as adjuvants in the treatment of cancer and other diseases in clinical practice under specific research protocols.

Interferon, another important biological response modifier, is now available as a prescription medicine. There are several varieties of interferon which can stimulate the immune system as well as slow down and even stop the growth of some cancer cells and of some viruses.Interleukins and tumor necrosis factors and BCG ore discussed elsewhere in the book

Included as BRM's are other substances whose mechanisms of action are poorly understood. These include BCG and C-Parvum vaccinations, and substances surrounded by mystique which, despite considerable controversy, are consistently reported to have distinct beneficial biological effects. The latter include 1) picibanil, 2) mistletoe, 3) Lentinan (a unique preparation from Japan)and other substances from mushrooms called glucans (e.g. "Maitake"), 4) Imuthiol (a preparation from the Merieux Institute in Paris), 5) vitamins A, E and C, and 6) Tufoin.

According to the published reports and presentations in BRM conferences, when these agents are used in combinations they appear to have a beneficial synergistic effect. Some enzyme preparations in combinations with other BRM's have been reported to be superior to either substance alone.

Advances in the understanding of enzymes

The modern age of enzymes started in the 20's with the development of ultracentrifugation by Svedberg, allowing separation of large molecules as well as enzymes. In 1926, Sumner crystallized urease, an enzyme that splits urea (like the enzyme in the urine that produces the known ammonia smell in the baby's diaper). Crystallization of other enzymes followed in the 1930's. In the 40's and 50's, modulation of all physiological reactions by enzymes was discovered. In 1960, the amino acid sequence of ribonuclease, an important cellular enzyme, was deduced. An important advance occurred in 1965 when X-ray crystallography was first used to demonstrate the three-dimensional structure of enzymes. Precise evaluations of the 3-D structure and amino acid sequence of enzymes was then possible. In 1969, the first chemical synthesis of an enzyme from amino acid precursors was reported. Recently, the application of recombinant DNA techniques has allowed the formation of 'designer enzymes' to accomplish specific tasks by inducing alterations ('mutations') at defined positions in the enzyme, thus altering the catalytic activity and specificity of the enzymes. Catalytic antibodies against stable components of enzymes were introduced recently to enhance the rate of the reactions. All of these and newer techniques have allowed more precise purification of enzymes. A significant advance has been the development of stabilization techniques to prevent enzyme degradation. These include encapsulation within a matrix such as within erythrocyte ghosts or liposomes, and cross linking to such other substances as antibodies. A number of additional but highly-technical advances have been reported but are beyond the scope of this book.

Enzymes for medical diagnosis

In the United States, the major importance of enzymes in medicine at present is in the measurement of enzyme levels as an aid to diagnosis. They are used to determine the level of specific enzymes present in the blood, urine, body fluids or tissues. Diagnostic enzymes are also important in estimating the concentrations of substrates or metabolites. Progress has been obtained in diagnosis because a wider variety of pure and stable enzymes, as noted before, are now commercially available. Also, highly sophisticated equipment and techniques are now available for enzyme assays. These include radioimmunoassays and enzyme immunoassays designed to measure the levels of specific enzymes. Many of these enzyme tests are easy to assay and automate. These tests are often preferred over older tests because they are highly reliable and reproducible, and because the differences between the normal specimen and the diseased specimen are clearly demonstrable and diagnostically significant. The enzymes utilized are sufficiently stable and allow storage for a limited but reasonable time. With these advances there has been a parallel increase in laboratory research utilizing similar sophisticated techniques and equipment.

Available diagnostic tests can demonstrate plasma-specific enzymes that are associated with the normal function of the plasma, such as blood coagulation components, complement activation components and lipoprotein metabolism. Newer tests can also determine nonplasma-specific enzymes, such as those resulting from abnormal cellular metabolism that have no actual function in the plasma where coenzymes or substrates are lacking. They are present in the plasma as a result of other body problems, such as liver disease, heart attacks, muscle diseases, diseases of the pancreas or cancer. Examples include some phosphatases, transaminases, lipases and amylases.

Current uses of enzymes in medicine

At present, in the United States and worldwide, certain specific medical enzymes are used legally as ethical and effective systemic treatments for a number of conditions. They are approved by the FDA for use in the treatment of specific diseases where there is general agreement about their effectiveness. These conditions or illnesses include: 1) cardiovascular disorders; 2) gastrointestinal conditions, particularly pancreatic insufficiency and related disorders; 3) replacement therapy of specific genetic disorders and deficiencies; 4) cancer treatment; 5) topical debridement of wounds (degradation of dying or necrotic tissue); and 6) removal of toxic substances from the blood.

In the United States, the 1993 Physicians Desk Reference (PDR) lists around 40 enzyme preparations approved by the FDA for use in this country. These include preparations for oral, injectable (intravenous or intramuscular use) or topical administration.

At present, the most publicized and probably most important therapeutic use of enzymes in the U.S. is in the treatment of various diseases where blood clots form and block blood vessels, producing serious problems. These are known as thromboembolic diseases. Included here are heart attacks (acute myocardial infarctions), blood clots of the legs and other areas (deep venous thrombosis), and blood clots in the lungs (extensive pulmonary embolism). They are also used for such related support services as for clogged arteriovenous canulae and for reperfusion. The enzymes used primarily for these purposes are *tissue plasminogen activator* (TPA), streptokinase and urokinase. The enzymes can be administered intracorporeally (intravascularly), or extracorporeally. The latter include various modalities of dialysis and pheresis. These will all be discussed in more detail later.

The treatment of gastrointestinal conditions with enzymes perhaps has been used the longest in medicine, and primarily utilizes orally administered medications. Commonly treated conditions include chronic pancreatic insufficiency, chronic pancreatitis, chronic fat intolerance (steatorrhea), and for replacement after removal of the pancreas (pancreatectomy). Most of the available preparations in the United States for these purposes are enzymes derived from the pig pancreas and are used singly or in variable combinations in different concentrations. These include amylase and proteases in dosages up to 180,000 USP units, and lipases from 5,000 to 25,000 USP units. Other specific enzymes are also used, such as lactase for disaecharidase deficiency, and sucrase-isomaltase for pancreatic insufficiency.

The treatment of *cystic fibrosis* (CF) is another important use of enzymes. Here, we have a genetic disorder affecting multiple organs, including the gastrointestinal system. The genetic defect involves a chloride transporting protein. CF occurs in 1 of 2,000 white and 1 of 17,000 black live births. The defect is present in a specific chromosome. It is characterized by chronic obstructive pulmonary disease, abnormally high sweat electrolytes and pancreatic insufficiency. The pancreas does not produce the enzymes necessary to break down the mucus of the lungs, thus preverting it from being dissolved normally. This results in the hyaline membrane disease of babies. The pancreatic insufficiency results in deficiency of the enzymes trypsin and lipase which in turn results in the loss of protein and fat in the feces with consequent malnutrition and growth retardation. The sweat abnormality helps doctors confirm the diagnosis by testing the levels of electrolytes. CF is treated with oral pancreatic enzyme mixtures as listed above. It also requires comprehensive nutritional and medical supportive measures and preventive treatment. This, however, is symptomatic treatment. At present, a number of research activities have centered around attempts to better delineate and then repair the

defective gene. Other approaches being investigated include iden-
tification of the missing enzyme and then trying to replace it.

Systemic enzyme replacement for various deficiency diseases is
the subject of intense research at present. Several such disorders
can be treated by practicing physicians but treatment for others is
only available in specific research medical centers where they are
being studied. Although a large number are under study, we will
mention only a few. One form of *severe combined immunodeficiency* (SCID) akin to the 'bubble boy disease' has been found to
be due to deficiency of the enzyme adenosine deaminase (ADA).
A commercial product under the trade name of Adagen$_{TM}$, containing pegademase, a source of ADA of bovine origin, is available
for intramuscular administration in patients who have failed bone
marrow transplants or who are considered poor candidates for
the same.

Phenylketonuria is a genetic disorder or inborn error of amino
acid metabolism characterized by the constant excretion of the
amino acid phenylalanine and its derivatives. It can result in mental retardation, seizures and other neurological problems. The
condition can be treated with the enzyme phenylalanine hydroxy-
lase. A specific form of emphysema known as congenital alpha-1
antitrypsin deficiency, a disease which produces chronic and progressive respiratory failure, can be treated with an enzyme known
as alpha-1 proteinase inhibitor or prolastin. Progress has also
been reported in the treatment with recombinant glucocerebro-
sides of Gaucher's disease, a disturbance of lipid metabolism
which produces severe enlargement of the spleen and liver, anemia, low platelets, low white cell count, bone changes, hemorrhage and brownish-ochre pigmentation of the skin and
conjunctivae of the eyes.

Enzyme treatments for cancer appear highly promising in medicine. The rationale includes blocking with enzymes the specific
amino acids in the serum that are required by a specific type of
cancer. Certain types of cancer appear to have lost the ability to
synthesize amino acids and are dependent on uptake of these

amino acids from the serum. Only those amino acids which are not the essential amino acids required by the body for life can be blocked. Normal cells can synthesize all but the eight (8) essential amino acids, so that the nonessential can be blocked as long as the essential are not disturbed.

At present, only one enzyme agent is listed in the U.S. Physicians Desk Reference (PDR) for use against cancer. This is the enzyme L-asparaginase, marketed under the trade name of Elspar. It is initially administered intravenously and subsequently intramuscularly. It is approved for use against *acute lymphocytic leukemia*, and is used primarily in combination with other chemotherapeutic agents in the treatment of children with this disease. It has also been used for *acute lymphoblastic leukemia* and *acute nonlymphoblastic leukemia*.

A number of other enzymes are currently under investigation for other forms of cancer. These include arginase, glutaminase, serine dehydratase, phenylalanine-ammonia lyase and leucine dehydrogenase. Still some other enzymes have been found to cause regression of lymphosarcomas in mice and some are known to delay other tumors in other animals.

Enzymes used in the United States for topical treatment of wounds or degradation of dying or necrotic tissue include the so-called debridement, fibrinolytic and collagenolytic enzyme mixtures. Debridement enzymes generally contain papain, trypsin, desoxyribonuclease or fibrinolysin in various combinations. Fibrinolytic enzymes contain combinations of the obove listed debridement enzymes as well as casein, lipase, amylase or protease. Collagenolytic enzymes contain collagenase.

The removal of toxic substances or undesired metabolites from the blood utilizing enzymes is often performed in combination with other procedures such as dialysis. Here, the blood is 'cleansed' of impurities by exposing it to the enzymes. The purified blood is then returned back to the patient.

In the U.S., most of the available oral preparations are either mixtures of cnzymes or single enzymes prescribed primarily for gastrointestinal disorders. A number of enzymes and enzyme mixtures are also available over-the-counter as digestive aids.

One specific oral proteolytic enzyme deserves specific mention since it is the only enzyme listed in the PDR as an orally administered anti-inflammatory enzyme medication approved for use in the U.S. It is listed in the PDR under the trade name "Bromase" and contains bromalein. The mechanism of action is listed as a 'prostaglandin modulator'. The treatment indications are listed as "inflammatory conditions resulting from prostaglandin metabolism, surgical procedures, sports activities, and other trauma."

Similar preparations have been available in Europe for around 40 years. The most frequently prescribed enzyme medications are the various proteolytic or hydrolytic enzyme mixtures. These include the original enzyme mixture developed in New York City by Drs. Wolf and Benitez. At present, these drugs are not approved for medical use in the United States, but one of the mixtures is the subject of an ongoing FDA approved clinical study. It has its own FDA IND (Investigational New Drug) number, a preliminary step before a drug can be considered for investigation and possible subsequent approval.

This brings us to the subject of orally administered enzymes for the treatment of inflammatory and other conditions.

Anti-inflammatory and oncologic uses of enzymes outside the U.S.

The use of therapeutic enzymes in Europe and other countries is similar to their use in the United States, with one exception. Oral proteolytic or hydrolytic enzyme mixtures are used more extensively as ethical, approved medical treatments outside the United States. Millions of patients are treated yearly with these preparations. In particular, they are frequently used in the treatment of arthritides, multiple sclerosis, autoimmune disorders and cancer. In reference to cancer, studies in Korea and Europe have reported an overall decrease in mortality and a decrease in relapse rates after oral therapeutic enzyme mixtures. An apparent decrease in mortality was also reported in Korea by a highly respected scientist and internationally recognized immunologist, Dr. Chin Po Kim, who cited a remarkable 23% overall five-year mortality rate in cancer patients who received oral enzyme mixtures. This compares very favorably with the results of the standard chemotherapy and radiation treatments cited in the American medical literature (DeVita).

This book reviews the clinical experiences and therapeutic results reported outside the United States after systemic hydrolytic enzyme treatments for various clinical conditions, with emphasis on long-term results.

Rationale for oral enzymes as a form of treatment

During the past 40 years, oral enzymes have been used in Europe and other countries as an approved, ethical and widely accepted modality of treatment for a variety of conditions. All of the conditions treated share a common denominator. In each one of these diseases, regardless of their cause, an uncontrolled inflammatory process occurs. This inflammation is associated with deposition of a blood clotting protein called fibrin at the tissue sites affected by each one of these diseases, and/or with formation of immune complexes. Of importance, all these diseases involve similarly deranged responses on the part of the various components of the immune system to their uncontrolled pathological processes. The published reports regarding the results of multiple clinical studies of treatments utilizing oral hydrolytic enzymes for a variety of medical conditions with similar immunopathology are indeed impressive. This is easier to understand if one realizes that, regardless of the cause, the human body has a rather specific and basic immunopathological response activated for all offenders. Therefore, a treatment directed at the basic immunopathological process makes considerable sense from a scientific point of view. Certainly it constitutes a most logical approach. An effective non toxic immune aiding drug against the basic immunopathologic charges would come close to the ideal form of treatment. Treatments with biological response modifiers (BRM's) and systemic enzymes follow this rationale and herald significant advances in this emerging treatment modality.

One should not be too surprised about a specific medication working for different clinical conditions since the world's most used drug, aspirin, also works for a variety of different conditions.

Of interest is the fact that this therapeutic approach with an orally administered mixture of enzymes was initially researched and developed in New York City by Dr. Max Wolf, then a researcher at Fordham and Columbia Universities. And yet, at present, this treatment modality is virtually unknown and therefore hardly used by practicing physicians in the United States. The authors have looked in great detail into the rationale and uses of this form of treatment. We were sufficiently impressed with the entire concept so that we felt a book on the subject was justified.

Can American medicine ignore a treatment modality that is at present prescribed legally, ethically and reportedly with great success to over 200,000 patients per year, including 70,000 cancer patients and 50,000 patients with vascular disorders? A treatment that has been administered to over 15 million patients during the past 15 years and which by all reports appears to be safer than most other modalities of treatment currently available for the same conditions?

We have asked ourselves, why is it that the enzyme treatments are unknown or not used by the United States medical establishment? A number of explanations have come to light and these will be discussed in the book. One of the principal reasons is 'traditional medical dogma'. It seems that malpractice concerns and the natural tendency of most American physicians to avoid appearing to espouse 'alternative' medicine to a large extent account for the inertia. In addition, American physicians tend to frown on treatments involving natural remedies which we often relegate to the somewhat 'separate' arenas of naturopathy, home-opathy or alternative medicine. Physicians in the U.S. basically have a justified reluctance to prescribe medications or treatments we may feel have not been scientifically proven in the United States. If it has not been researched in the U.S., it is unlikely that a drug will be approved by the Food and Drug Administration. Likewise, in order for a drug to be approved, research conducted in the U.S. is required. Research from other countries alone is seldom, if ever, accepted for FDA approval. Research is very expensive and unless it is sponsored at a university medical center or by the National Institutes of Health or one of the giant pharmaceutical corporations, chances of adequate research being conducted in the U.S. are poor. Because of various reasons mentioned, including the prevailing impression that 'a treatment which is not used in the U.S. does not work', the various NIH or university scientists who generally apply for research grants have shown little interest in oral therapeutic enzyme research. Another aspect illustrating physician reluctance is that a number of unrelated enzyme products are currently available in the U.S. as over-the-counter preparations, and most physicians will not recommend products they may equate with OTC preparations, even if they are found to be effective, in part for fear of being labeled unscientific because the patients that go to see the doctor expect 'a real prescription or injection'. The prevailing medical opinion is that patients should be treated exclusively with FDA approved 'real' medications.

A significant development, according to reports in the media, is that the U.S. federal government has recently announced a new scientific division to investigate some of the so-called 'alternative therapies'. In addition, an FDA approved clinical study utilizing a mixture of oral enzymes is currently in progress in the U.S.

Purported mechanism of action

The European pharmacological and medical literature cites the mechanisms of action of oral hydrolytic enzymes as fibrinolytic, antiedematous, anti-inflammatory and analgesic effects. They are also felt to stimulate the elimination of submetabolites, debris and toxins via the activation of the mononuclear phagocyte system (MPS). They were felt to have a selective anticancer cell activity (selective oncocytolysis) causing cancer cells to loose their nuclei, substantially disintegrate and finally progress to complete cell destruction or cytolysis. Studies also reported that proteolytic enzymes activated macrophages and natural killer (NK) cells by breaking down immune complexes which block these cells (Figure 4 and 5). Other reports revealed that they are also thought to induce release of beneficial mediators required for proper inflammation control, including the powerful and very important tumor necrosis factor alpha (TNF-α), and the mediators interleukin 1-β and interleukin 6.

Tumor necrosis factor (TNF) deserves further comment because of its great importance in protecting us, and its potential use for treatment. This cytokine, also known as TNF-α or cachectin, is a polypeptide. It is produced and released by scavenger cells (macrophages) or their precursors, the peripheral blood mononuclear cells (PBMC), in our bodies. It can be purified from tissue culture supernatants or produced in larger quantities by biotechnology companies as a recombinant form of human (hTNF-α) origin. This is obtained from human serum or from tissue culture supernatants containing the natural or native human TNF and utilizing recombinant techniques. For laboratory studies, murine sources are also utilized (mTNF-α).

Recent studies have demonstrated that TNF occurs in the body as an active and an inactive form. Activation, to a large extent, appears to be determined by two types of cell markers: Small and large cell receptors. The smaller receptors are present in most cells and allow TNF to induce cytotoxicity when needed. The larger receptors are present only in certain lymphoid cells, particularly the so-called 'T' and 'B' cells. In certain animal studies, these larger receptors do not bind to the circulating TNF. This activated TNF or 'cachectin' is felt to be responsible for the biologic activity and, when in excess, systemic toxicity. Mutant forms of TNF have been developed which can express a higher level of the desired cytotoxicity with a reduced level of systemic toxic effects. These are under study for eventual human use. The denatured, inactive TNF is felt to be composed of a smaller polypeptide unit called a monomer. The natural, activated TNF is felt to be composed of combinations of polypeptides forming more complex and higher molecular weight structures called dimers or trimers.

TNF-α functions by interacting with special high affinity receptors on the cells. The receptors mediate internalization of the TNF which leads to its biological actions. Its main functions include growth regulatory responses (Smith & Baglioni) and breakdown of unwanted cells (cytotoxity), thus leading to tumor necrosis. Unfortunately, under certain conditions like terminal cancer or AIDS, excessive amounts of this TNF agent are released into the circulation in an abortive attempt to destroy the offending cells. This results in, or contributes to, a number of ill effects such as marked weight loss, wasting, fever, malaise, etc., a condition generally designated as cachexia.

According to Ostade et al, TNF has a remarkable ability to selectively kill or inhibit malignant cell lines in laboratory studies, especially when used in combination with interferon. This ability is so far unmatched by any other combinations of cytokines. However, clinical trials in cancer patients have on the whole been disappointing. It is felt that TNF and other cytokines polymerize at high serum concentrations, causing them to lose their tumoricidal effect. The hydrolytic/proteolytic enzymes are felt to be able to cleave the polymerized TNF and interleukin (IL) derivatives allowing them to regain their tumoricidal activity. Selective destruction of tumor cells with liquefaction ('colliquative or coagulative necrosis' or oncocytolysis) has also been reported by others.

Leskovar reported that preliminary treatment with proteolytic enzymes increased the activity of macrophages up to 700%, and that of natural killer (NK) cells up to 1,300% within a short period of time after administration.

Desser reported that proteolytic enzymes stimulate the peripheral blood mononuclear cells (PBMC), which include the circulating precursors of the scavenger cells or macrophages, to produce TNF. A dose-dependent, increased formation of the 'good' TNF-α by these cells is felt to occur. Enzymes have also been reported to stimulate the same cells (PBMC) to produce other cytokines, including interleukin 1 and interleukin 6. The proteases can have a regulatory effect by their interaction with the antiproteases (α-2M, α1-antitrypsin), which in turn react with the cytokine derivatives (TNF, IL).

A separate action of oral hydrolytic enzymes involving increased penetration of medications into connective tissue has also been reported separately by Chain, Sanella and Hechter. They are felt to enhance the absorption and effects of such concomitantly administered medications as antibiotics and anticancer cytotoxic drugs. This is reported to apply also to tissues where the focus is difficult to reach, such as the paranasal sinuses, prostate, scar tissues, etc. (Barsom et al., Baumgartner).

A fibrinolytic action of enzymes was reported as "dissolution of fibrin and fibrin mantles thus limiting clot formation, reducing the blood viscosity and improving the circulation" (Nakahara, Purcell, Inderst). Oral hydrolytic enzymes also were reported to 'allow the red blood cells to alter their shape so that they can adapt their form in order to pass through the finest capillary vessels', thus functioning in a more normal fashion and improving the microcirculation (Inderst, Maehder, Mörl).

The anti-inflammatory effect of oral hydrolytic/proteolytic enzymes is felt to be quite complex and to involve several different mechanisms. The action has been explained primarily by their action on immune complexes. This was felt to be brought about by enzymatic cleavage of a component (Fc fragment) of the immunoglobulin portion, in part mediated through the modulation of its surface markers. Hydrolytic enzymes were also felt to be able to reduce the damaging effect of the complement cascade, itself the 'killer enzyme cascade' of the normal immune system (Figure 1). In addition, reports from other studies indicated that the proteolytic enzymes are felt to detach or separate important receptors called 'adhesion molecules' which are responsible for the adhesion or anchoring of undesirable molecules and cells to normal blood vessel walls and other tissue membranes (Kleine, Mahr, Yamoda).

Clinical studies worldwide

During the past 40 years, numerous scientific studies and clinical evaluations of the use of oral hydrolytic enzymes for various medical conditions have been conducted worldwide. These are reviewed in this book. In addition, the Enzyme Research Institute reports over 150 clinical and scientific studies presently in progress at different medical centers worldwide.

Legal issues

At the present time, oral hydrolytic enzymes are approved in a number of European countries, Mexico and in some countries in South America for use in the treatment of various diseases reviewed in this book. Other oral enzymes are approved in Japan for use in a variety of medical conditions. In the United States, approved uses of enzymes have already been listed. Oral proteolytic enzymes are currently the subject of clinical evaluations. Some hydrolytic enzyme preparations are available as 'digestive supplements' in health food stores, but these are not approved at present for treatment of any other conditions.

Controversies surrounding the use of oral hydrolytic enzymes

The main controversy regarding oral hydrolytic or proteolytic enzymes can be best summarize in one word: Absorption. For this reason, absorption will be discussed in more detail below (see page 27).

Controversy dates back to the origin of medical enzymes for treatment. Some of the early investigators obtained excellent clinical results while others could not duplicate or confirm the same. Enzyme researchers point out the discrepancy was due to the fact that fresh materials of animal or plant origin appeared to have an effect, although the activity ceased the moment the enzymes were denatured by aging or heat. Unfortunately, the idea that they did not work persisted and became dogma, even though according to the published reports, the lack of effect was due to the administration of inactive preparations.

A recent presentation at a national Biological Response Modifier Symposium in Tulsa, Oklahoma, stressed some of the controversies regarding oral enzymes (Larrick). These controversies will be discussed in some detail since they underscore the concerns and opinions frequently mentioned regarding the use of hydrolytic or proteolytic enzymes.

The presenter (Dr. Larrick) reviewed some of the oral enzyme preparations available in Europe for oral adjuvant therapy of cancer and other diseases. He also reviewed some of the studies purported to demonstrate efficacy in cancer, various rheumatologic conditions and AIDS.

Doubts were expressed regarding the hypothesis that enzymes work due to the elimination of immune complexes. This presentation did not appear to specifically dispute the clinical effectiveness of oral enzymes. Instead, it was suggested that their effect may be due to the enzymes acting by

1)   the generation of exorphins;

2)   the results of quercetin (rutin) used in the preparations;

3)   an action on the pancreas; or

4)   a placebo effect.

It was also mentioned that one patient reported by a Dutch group using an injectable preparation containing an enzyme mixture developed circulatory shock immediately after the injection in spite of the purported high degree of safety of adjuvant enzymes, casting doubts about their safety. Finally, some questions were raised regarding the enteric absorption of enzymes.

We looked at these issues and reviewed the pertinent medical literature. The following represents a summary of our findings.

Absorption

An interesting indication of absorption of orally administered hydrolytic enzymes was first noted by Dr. Max Wolf, the pioneering physician often regarded as the 'father of enzymes'. His biography is reviewed in the book (Chapter 7, p. 114). Dr. Wolf injected indigo blue dye into the skin of the backs of laboratory animals, creating a dime-sized blue spot. He then administered oral placebo and the spot showed little change. When he administered oral hydrolytic enzymes the blue spot site would spread to cover the entire back of the animal within the first 2 to 3 hours after administration. He was impressed by this finding and inspired to continue his research. Because the techniques available at the time could not properly confirm absorption into the blood circulation or lymphatics, emphasis was placed on demonstration of pharmacological and clinical effects. In recent years, absorption has been studied in more detail.

Because of their large molecular size, enzymes are regarded as macromolecules. The absorption of intact macromolecules, including enzymes, was thought to be impossible for years. With the availability of highly specific methods of analysis, it has become possible to study the absorption of enzymes and other macromolecular proteins from the gut into the blood and/or lymphatics. Although several methods are available to study the absorption of enzymes, radiochromatographic measurements and immunofluorescent techniques appear highly reliable. The pharmacological effect of the macromolecules can also be studied qualitatively and scientifically. However, actual quantitative measurement of these macromolecules is most difficult because of a variety of factors, such as competing internal body enzymes (hydrolases), antiprotease interference (body substances which react with the enzymes masking their detection) and redistribution of the administered enzymes.

Reports of studies utilizing different techniques have indicated that orally administered hydrolytic enzymes are absorbed in a manner similar to the 'enteropancreatic circulation'. The latter is generally accepted as the mechanism responsible for the reabsorption of pancreatic enzymes from the gut into the circulation and then back into the pancreas.

Three mechanisms have been suggested for the absorption of the intact molecules of orally administered hydrolytic enzymes. These include: 1) transcellular absorption through the mucosal epithelial cells followed by a process called pinocytosis; 2) entrapment by alpha-2 macroglobulin protein inhibitor (α-2M) or by alpha-1 antiprotease and then absorption into the lymphatics; and 3) transcellular absorption via the gut-associated immune system at the level of the Peyer's patches and solitary follicles (Figures 2 and 3).

It has also been reported that only a portion of the orally administered enzymes are absorbed intact via the above listed mechanisms. Published studies have indicated that from 10 to 40% of the oral hydrolytic enzyme mixture administered is absorbed (Menzel et al., Steffen et al., Seifert et al., Felix, Kleine). It is assumed that a larger percentage, from 60 to 90% of the enzyme macromolecules, are broken down into amino acid chains and peptide components and then absorbed.

Menzel et al., Steffen et al. and Seifert et al. verified absorption of isotope labeled enzymes (hydrolases) from the G.I. tract of rabbits, guinea pigs and rats. According to Professor G. Gerbert, a

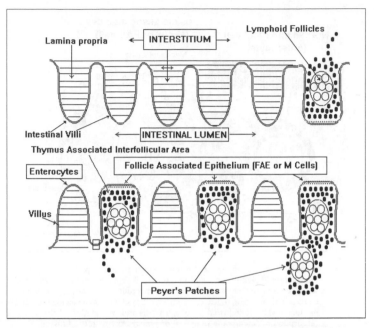

Figure 2: Schematic representation of gut-associated immune system with Peyer's patches containing lymphoid follicles, thymus-associated areas and follicle associated epithelium [FAE or M (membranous) cells]

physiologist at the University of Ulm, the intestinal epithelium which has been thought to be impermeable to larger molecules can be crossed by macromolecules, including intact proteins. Macromolecules normally penetrate the mucosal surface via the transcellular route (Figure 3), since the intercellular bridges (tight junctions) between the enterocytes prohibit free intercellular or paracellular passage. The macromolecule binds to the enterocyte cell membrane facing the intestinal lumen. This is followed by phagocytosis with entrapment of the macromolecular material within pinched off fragments of the cellular membrane via a pro-

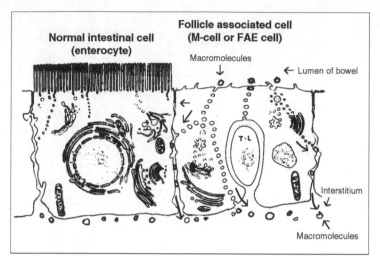

Figure 3: Schematic representation of the transcellular transport pathways across the intestinal epithelium. A normal intestinal cell or enterocyte is shown on the left. According to Gebert and others, such macromolecules as enzymes come in contact with and bind to the enterocyte's cell wall membrane facing the intestinal lumen. This is followed by phagocytosis and vesiculation of the material (absorption by 'membrane pinching' or pinocytosis) with the subsequent production of phagosomes. Some of these, in turn, bind with some of the cell's own enzyme packets (lysosomes) to produce phagolysosomes where the macromolecules may be broken down further into smaller components. However, other macromolecules escape intracellular digestion and are extruded through the basolateral membrane (the cell walls on the sides) from where they enter the interstitial space below the mucosa and may be taken up by macrophages and lymphoid cells. Those macromolecules not taken up by these cells eventually escape into the blood or lymph. This transport is much faster at the sites of the so-called 'gut-associated immune system' which is composed of lymphoid cells. These cells are found in specialized structures of the intestine known as the *Peyer's patches* or as solitary aggregates of lymphoid cells known as *follicles*. Both of these structures contain specialized intestinal cells known as the *follicular associated enterocytes* (FAE) which are also known as *membranous cells, microfold containing* cells or *M-cells* (shown on the right in). They have been seen to allow a more efficient and faster transport of macromolecules. In the M-cell noted on the right, the enzyme containing vesicles (phagolysosomes) are depicted as small circles. T-L represents a T-cell type of lymphocyte. Current research supports functional transfer of intact enzyme macromolecules into the circulation via the above noted mechanism. Once in the circulation, they are bound to such antiproteinases as alpha-2 macroglobulin and alpha-1 antiproteinase. From here, researchers postulate that they are released at sites of inflammation.

cess of vesiculation known as pinocytosis. Some of the vesicles formed fuse with specialized intracellular enzyme packets called lysosomes, and some of the macromolecular proteins and peptides may be hydrolyzed by lysosomal enzymes within the resulting phagolysosomes. Other macromolecules escape intracellular digestion, are extruded through the basal membrane into the underlying interstitial connective tissue area, and are released from their entrapment within the pinocytic membrane or vesicle. In the interstitial space, the macromolecules become available to macrophages and lymphoid cells. Those not taken up by these cells, possibly still within pinocytic vesicles, eventually escape into the blood or lymph.

The efficiency of the transfer of macromolecular material from the lumen of the bowel to the submucosal areas (interstitium) is pronounced in the epithelium covering lymphoid structures like Peyer's patches or solitary follicles, which are the principal components of the gut associated immune system (Figures 2 and 3). In particular, the Peyer's patches are most interesting since they are felt to actively 'open and close' in response to proteins coming in contact with their centers. In these regions, specialized mucosal cells or enterocytes, the FAE (follicle associated epithelium) or M-cells (a designation based on the occurrence of 'microfolds' facing the gut lumen and their 'membranous' appearance) are felt to convey macromolecular material in both directions – from gut into lymphatics and vice versa. Thus, this gut-associated immune system is supplied with potentially antigenic macromolecules from the intestinal lumen, some of which are then 'neutralized' and transported into the lymphatics while others are inactivated at the site and presented for destruction. Likewise, the plasma cells present in the submucosal connective tissue area called the lamina propria produce immunoglobulins, particularly IgA. The latter is considered the mucosal defense patrol. These IgA molecules are transported transcellularly to the epithelial surface on the intestinal lumen where they protect us from allergy-inducing food proteins and other substances.

The extent of the intestinal absorption of intact molecules or large breakdown products of food proteins, including dietary enzymes, is not yet clarified. According to Professor Gebert, although it had been generally assumed that almost all of the dietary protein is split into amino acids or small peptides before it is absorbed by the mucosa, some experimental results support the hypothesis that a greater part of dietary protein is taken up in the form of macromolecules and that the final step of splitting into amino acids takes place in the peripheral tissues ('distributed digestion').

The intestinal transport of macromolecules is especially important for the fate of digestive enzymes. Hydrolases like trypsin or elastase can be taken up and transferred functionally intact into the circulation. They can be reabsorbed from the bloodstream by the pancreatic cells (enteropancreatic circulation) as a conservation mechanism. The circulating proteases are bound to antiproteases like alpha-2 macroglobulin or alpha-1 antiprotease. Thus, the intestinal absorption of intact enzymes might be important for the balance between hydrolases and antiproteases in the extracellular space, an important factor for the stabilization of the internal *milieu* of the organism.

Regardless of its nutritional significance, the transepithelial transfer of particulate matter is at least antigenically sufficient to elicit a response of the gut-associated immune system, and the production and secretion of the respective immunoglobulins promote binding and proteolysis of the antigenic materials on the mucosal brush-border, thereby reducing their absorption (immunological barrier).

A system of very important defense and carrier proteins within our bodies called antiproteases has been described in detail. Recent reports have described the function and mode of action of these protease inhibitors in our serum. The two most important antiproteases are called alpha-1 antitrypsin (AAT) and alpha-2 macroglobulin (α-2M). In addition to transport they maintain the body´s equilibrium between macromolecules and macroglobulins.

Their main known functions involve binding to proteases (enzymes) and to cytokines (cellular immune mediations). If we compare the enzymes to soldiers, the antiproteases then represent amphibious armed personnel carriers. They enclose and carry the proteases to their final destination, whether it would be for their destruction or for a necessary body function. The alpha-1 antitrypsin reacts with trypsin and chymotrypsin, inactivating their enzymatic activity. On the other hand, the alpha-2 macroglobulin forms an enzymatically active complex with the proteases or with cytokines, and together they become 'activated' and react with a specific target such as the cells of the mononuclear phagocyte system (MPS). According to Adams, for example, high titers of free or inactive α-2M inhibit the endogenous proteases and the tumor destroying capabilities of the MPS. Thus, it is thought that binding to proteases (such as the administered therapeutic enzymes) would have a beneficial effect by lowering the titers of the inactive and free α-2M.

Recent studies also demonstrate the second important immunological effects of the 'activated α-2M complex'. They are very important in the transport and distribution of essential cellular substances called cytokines which function as immune agents or mediators. The α-2M also forms 'activated complexes' with these cytokines, and transports them from the intravascular into the extravascular space where they are needed. For example, the cytokines known as tumor necrosis factor (TNF) are very important in a number of diseases. They are produced in two forms, a 'good TNF' and a 'bad TNF'. These native and altered TNF forms are regulated by the α-2M. Thus, TNF-alpha has a higher affinity for the α-2M complex. This is also true of another cytokine known as interleukin-1beta (IL-1ß). Other cytokines, like IL-6, bind preferentially to the unchanged free α-2M. Those cytokines bound to the 'activated α-2M complex' are themselves inactivated and eliminated rapidly. Since excess of these cytokines can have a negative effect in some instances (TNF-alpha and IL-1beta), it appears that the activated α-2M complex plays a beneficial role.

It has been reported that some macromolecules such as orally administered enzymes come in contact with the gut-associated immune system and are actually bound by these antiproteases. The antiproteases are felt to 'surround and wrap themselves around the macromolecules. By so doing, the antiproteases can prevent antigenicity, thus preventing allergic and anaphylactic reactions, according to Starkey et al, Miyata et al, Travis et al and Kleine. Their role in macromolecular absorption at the level of the enterocyte cell surface is the subject of current studies and requires further confirmation.

If absorbed, do they remain intact in the blood? Are they inactivated by protease inhibitors? Are they broken down?

It has been furthermore suggested by Larrick that, "if and once the enzymes are absorbed they are promptly inactivated in the serum by the protease inhibitors." The latter are naturally occurring macromolecules present in our bodies, particularly in the serum. They have been estimated to comprise around 10% of the total volume of all plasma proteins. Some of the protease inhibitors were discussed in the previous section. Their function in the body is not fully understood, but they are regarded as important in several ways and probably essential to life. They are important in the transport and modulation of other plasma proteins, including proteases, cytokines, and possibly immunoglobulins. A partial list of the protease inhibitors includes alpha-2 macroglobulin (α-2M), alpha-2 plasmin inhibitor, alpha-1 antitrypsin, 'C-1 prime inhibitor' component of complement, antithrombin III, etc. We have emphasized α-2M because it appears to be the prototype of this group of substances.

Recent reports by LaMarre et al, and by Heumann & Vischer have shed some light into the function of these macroglobulins. α-2M is a large glycoprotein present in high concentrations in human plasma (2 to 3.5 GM/liter). Major sources of α-2M are the liver cells, macrophages and fibroblasts. The liver cells and macrophages are also responsible for the clearance of the α-2M. The macrophage and fibroblast production explains the presence of α-2M in the tissues and in tumors. Two forms have been described, native and activated α-2M. The major functions of α-2M are its non-specific, protease-binding capacity and its more recently recognized cytokine-binding activity. Before we explain these actions, let us digress to look at the cytokines. These are substances generated by our cells and are composed of small polypeptides. They initiate responses in other cells by interacting with specific cell surface receptors. Included here are the interleukins, interferons, growth factors, tumor necrosis factor, etc. Some of these also have enzymatic properties. They are important in inflammation and tissue repair, and some demonstrate hormonal activity. When produced in excess or inappropriately, they are associated with chronic inflammation and with such diseases as pulmonary fibrosis, glomerulonephritis, cachexia in malignancies or AIDS, etc. Therefore, any methods of controlling excessive or inappropriate cytokine activity may have a beneficial effect in these diseases. It is felt that α-2M modulates cytokines and may thus have a beneficial effect in inflammatory conditions.

The function of α-2M as an antiprotease has been studied extensively. According to the 'trap hypothesis', the targeted protease initiates an 'encounter' with the native α-2M and enzymatically cleaves a specific peptide bond within the center or 'bait' area of the α-2M. The latter then undergoes conformational changes trapping the protease inside and forming a nondissociable complex. This conformational complex is called the activated α-2M. According to the studies of LaMarre and others, the important thing to remember is that these activated complexes retain their enzymatic activity and are capable of interacting with small substrates which can penetrate into the enzyme's (protease's) 'active site'. Thus, although the antiproteases bind and wrap themselves around the enzymes, the latter remain active and the α-2M functions more like a modulating and transport vehicle. This can be compared to a soldier inside a tank who can still maneuver the tank and fire the weapons but cannot get out until the hatch is open and may be destroyed at a given time in the process. The enzymes in this activated complex state cannot be easily demonstrated by ordinary techniques, but their action is demonstrable. It appears that documentation of dose-related enzyme action therefore indirectly confirms their presence in the serum.

Do hydrolytic enzymes eliminate immune complexes?

It has been consistently proposed by the enzyme scientists that one of the major mechanisms of action of orally administered and systemically absorbed enzymes is to break down the immune complexes. This 'immune clearance' degrades the pathological immune complexes. Thus, this allows the macrophages to clear the breakdown products away, therefore allowing the body's immune defenses again to function more effectively against the aggressor, whether a cancerous cell or one of the other causes of inflammation.

Let's pause and look at these events in more detail. When a foreign substance enters the body, such as the protein from a microbe, that potential offender, called an antigen, can elicit a response from our immune defenses. The cells from the immune system conducting their normal surveillance will detect the antigen and then create and release immunoglobulins generally called antibodies to go and confront the antigen like policemen in 'hand-to-hand combat'. If enough of these antigens are present and enough antibodies are formed, in a sense they hold hands together and form a larger molecule composed of a variable number of antigens and antibodies. These are known as immune complexes. Under normal conditions, the antigen-antibody complexes are important in the recognition and elimination of such potentially dangerous structures as bacteria, viruses, fungi, toxins, cellular debris, early cancerous cells, etc. They then immobilize the unwanted particles, and stimulate the body's scavenger cells or macrophages and their precursor relatives, the monocytes, to immobilize, swallow, take away and destroy the offenders. Although immune complexes in proper amounts are initially helpful, particularly at the local tissue level where they become fixed, in excess quantities they overflow into the circulation and can then block other functions of the immune system and produce problems.

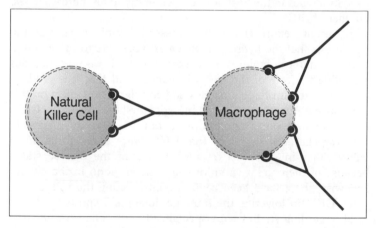

Figure 4:   Functions of immunoglobulins. The Y-shaped immunoglobulins (antibodies) are attracted to antigen receptors on the cell surfaces and activate these cells to perform their functions. If excessive, they can have a blocking effect.

During the past two decades, numerous articles in the scientific literature have reported clinical and laboratory studies documenting the presence of circulating immune complexes (CIC's) (Figures 4, 5 and 6) in autoimmune diseases, inflammatory disorders and cancer. In a number of instances, the level of CIC's have been correlated with the activity of the clinical illness. Other studies have documented a drop in CIC's following various forms of medical treatments, including orally administered enzyme mixtures. These studies have also documented clinical improvements when the CIC levels drop.

Increased levels of CIC have also been reported to have a significant detrimental role in cancer by blocking the body's own defenses. They are thought to be formed by the continuing stimulation of the immune system as cancers grow and thus constantly replace the antigens which are eliminated. These in turn lead to new antibodies in the host, and subsequently to an increase in the number of CIC's.

A recent report (Larrick) expressed doubts regarding the hypothesis that the hydrolytic enzymes work due to the elimination of immune complexes. It suggested that there is no consensus regarding the role of the CIC's in cancer and that it is unlikely that orally administered enzymes had any significant effect on this mechanism. According to some investigators, the role of the CIC's in cancer and other conditions is not as clear as suggested. Dobryszycka et al suggested that CIC's were found to be of no value either in diagnosis or surveillance of the disease status because of their 'great variations in concentration in the serum'. Likewise, there have been reports contradicting the role of elevated CIC's in lowering the immune defenses. Reports by Burgis et al. regarding studies with specialized cells called *lymphokine activated killer* (LAK) cells and by Nielsen et al. regarding natural killer (NK) cells (both of them important in the destruction of cancer) support this concept. Other reports dispute the concept that new antigens in cancer result in the formation of CIC's (Buch et al.), that CIC's fluctuate with disease status (Runowicz et al.), or that relapses (Laffaioli et al.) and metastases (Buch et al.) correlate with the level of CIC's.

On the other hand, the medical literature strongly supports the concept that CIC's are largely responsible for the cancer associated immunosuppression. Attempts at removal of the CIC's which block the body's defenses with various treatment modalities have been employed to reverse the immunosuppression. Although

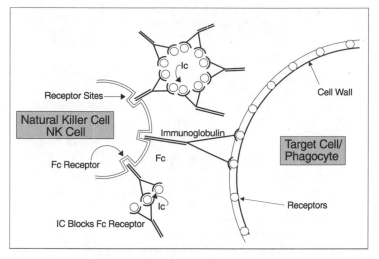

Figure 5: Immune complexes (y shoped aggregates). Immune reaction between killer cell and target cell mediated by antibody complexes. The natural killer cell cannot work properly because it is blocked by the immune complexes.

treatment with some of these agents have been effective in laboratory animals and in a few cancer patients, reduction of the CIC levels in some studies involving humans did not alter the course of the disease.

Contrary to the above cited negative reports, the proponents of therapeutic hydrolytic enzymes postulate that they basically disagree with the above cited conclusions based on the fact that these studies have primarily looked at circulating immune complexes. These enzyme scientists emphasize that the actual effect of the enzymes is on the tissue-bound immune complexes (TBIC's) and their surrounding fibrin mantle present at the actual sites of the inflammation or the cancer (Figures 5 and 6). They propose that it is only after treatment over a prolonged period of time that more and more of the TBIC's are reduced sufficiently also to

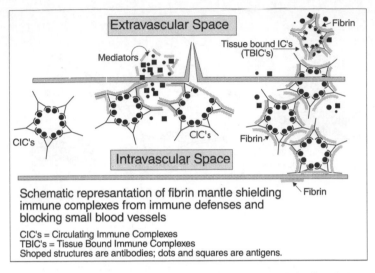

Figure 6:   Immune complexes in blood vessel adhere to endothelial cells and stimulate fibrin formation.

reduce the excess of other immune complexes circulating in the blood.

How safe are oral hydrolytic enzymes?

Clinical researchers and physicians using oral hydrolytic or proteolytic enzymes usually emphasize the relative freedom from serious side effects found after administration of these compounds. According to many physicians and clinical investigators experienced in the use of oral hydrolytic enzymes, and to patients, the enzymes are exceptionally well-tolerated. The side effects generally noted are quite mild and include mild gastrointestinal irritation, such as intestinal bloating, loose bowels, peculiar acrid smell of the stool and, in some cases, itching of the perianal area. Some patients noted mild sedation, loss of appetite and weight loss. No serious or life-threatening problems have been observed after the oral preparations. Rare allergic reactions have been noted after injectable preparations and after administration via enemas. One patient reported by a Dutch group (De Smet) was treated with an injectable preparation containing an enzyme mixture. It was reported that the patient developed circulatory shock immediately after the injection and this was interpreted as an allergic reaction to the enzyme mixture. Subsequent evaluation of this incident raised doubts as to the enzymes having caused the reaction and instead incriminated the use of procaine administered with the enzyme mixture. The patient reportedly refused to participate in a comprehensive evaluation by an allergist and the issue was not resolved any further.

Extensive toxicological studies have been conducted. No median lethal dose (LD_{50}) could be determined when given by mouth. No teratogenic, mutagenic or carcinogenic effects were noted at dosages substantially higher than the standard therapeutic dosages.

Generation of exorphins?

Opioids acting in our bodies can be of two types, endorphins and exorphins. Endorphins are endogenous morphine-like substances. They are substances which occur naturally in the body and can be generated or induced by various stimuli, such as heavy and persistent exercise, positive and enjoyable emotions or sexual excitement. Exorphins are externally administered or exogenous morphine-like substances, generally present in the diet.

Exorphins have been described as "peptide and protein fragments which bind to opioid receptors in our cells and mediate a number of important biological effects." They are generated in vivo during normal digestion. The generation of exorphins may explain the immense pleasure felt after eating certain types of foods, such as chocolate. Because they resemble opiates in their action, they have been called opioids. Since they bind to these opioid receptors they have morphine-like effects. They can produce analgesia, drowsiness, respiratory depression, reduced G.I. motility, or have anti-nausea, anti-emetic, anti-proliferative and enhanced cytotoxic activity.

Examples of these include exorphins present in milk or in gluten, the major protein in wheat germ. Casorphins are exorphins derived from proteins in the milk. It has been speculated that casorphins in the mother's milk are responsible for the child-mother bonding. Normally casorphins slow down the transit time of the bowel, allowing increased absorption of ingested foods or medications, possibly through a direct action on the brain. Some types of casorphins have been incriminated in the *sudden infant death syndrome* or SIDS.

It has also been suggested that exorphins may have activity in adjuvant cancer therapy because, as opioid agonists, they have anti-proliferative effects, increase the sense of well-being and synergize with other medications.

Our review does not contradict the previously expressed hypothesis regarding the induction of exorphins by oral hydrolytic enzymes. We accept this as a potential explanation for the beneficial effects of oral enzymes, worthy of study. However, our review suggests that other mechanisms also play a role. These are discussed under mechanism of action.

A rutin effect?

We do not think that the results of quercetin (rutin) used in the enzyme mixtures explains their action since rutin is present in only some of the preparations and the other mixtures lacking rutin have been reported to have an effect as good or better than those with rutin. However, more studies on quercetin alone would be justified to better elucidate the isolated effect of this one component.

Promote better digestion and absorption of essential nutrients?

Indeed, there is a likelihood that better digestion and absorption may be additional ways in which oral enzymes induce some of the clinically observed effects. Better absorption of essential vitamins, minerals, trace elements, fatty acids and nutrients translates into a better supply, and thus into a more efficient and healthier body. These nutrients are essential for all our functions, including metabolism, circulation of the immune and vascular systems, the repair system and even catabolism.

However, it is our feeling that this does not fully explain all of the enzyme effects since experimental intravenous, intralesional or intratumoral enzymes have also demonstrated significant and beneficial clinical effects.

Action of the pancreas?

An action on the pancreas was suggested based on studies where orally-administered proteases suppressed the exocrine pancreas and the cholecytokinin release. It was not explained how suppression of the exocrine pancreas can have anti-inflammatory or cell-suppressive effects. Studies published by Dr. Edward Howell in his book on enzymes suggests that when the pancreas has to work less as a result of proper and natural diets, the basic amino acid chains otherwise required by the pancreas for dietary uses are made available to the metabolic enzymes which are needed for every day health. Dr. Howell indicated that enzymes present in food are routinely destroyed by cooking and a diet without enzymes results in enlargement of the pancreas, with an increase in chronic degenerative diseases and cancer. He showed that when fresh or raw foods rich in enzymes are given in the diet enlargement of the pancreas was inhibited. He correlated the absence of pancreatic enlargement with a reduction in the incidence of chronic degenerative diseases and cancer.

Placebo effect?

Placebo effect is difficult to accept because anti-inflammatory effects of the enzyme mixtures have been demonstrated in laboratory animals by several independent investigators. Studies by Lindner and Forster, and more recently by Herrera, demonstrated reduction in artificially induced edema of the paws of laboratory animals when the enzyme mixtures as well as the individual enzymes were administered. These anti-inflammatory changes were dose-related. The higher the dose, the more the edema was reduced. Moreover, many recent clinical trials demonstrating anti-inflammatory response have included a control group receiving a placebo. The control group did not reveal any anti-inflammatory effects.

Authors comment about this book

During the past three decades, scientists have tried to learn more about enzymes and considerable progress has been attained. Due to the immense importance of enzymes to our bodies and to our health, and recognizing an increasing number of enzyme deficiencies as well as errors and interferences with our enzyme functions, research has led to remarkable advances in the understanding of enzyme systems. Scientists have studied how enzymes change in health and disease, and how to measure them in the blood, urine, body secretions and tissues for early diagnosis of diseases. During the past several years, there has also been an intense effort to use enzymes as treatments for correction of enzyme deficiencies or malfunctions, and for prevention of diseases. It is our purpose to review these advances and present them in this book to make the reader aware of this wonderfully fascinating and extremely important dimension of our health. A system which in our opinion has been the 'abandoned and neglected child of medicine'. Even the United States has lagged behind in enzyme research, primarily due to 'previous dogma' that minimizes their importance, and to confusion and contradiction in the American medical literature regarding their status.

This book deals with the various aspects of enzymes in medicine and health, and presents an overview of the subject. Our goal is to bring an understanding and awareness of the advances in this field to the attention of the American public. We emphasize their importance in every one's health and hope to generate more interest which will lead to more research in the United States regarding the medical aspects of this vital system of our bodies.

In this book, we also review various systemic enzyme treatments used in Europe, Japan and other countries, but currently not used in the United States. Although approved in other countries, some of the treatments are not approved by the FDA for use in the U.S. at the present time. It should be clearly understood from the beginning that our review does not constitute an endorsement of specific treatments, a guide to self diagnosis or self treatment or a medical recommendation for their indiscriminate use. All readers are urged to contact their family or personal physicians for specific medical problems. It is not our purpose to recommend enzymes for any specific conditions for which they are not medically indicated in the United States. We feel that any medical treatments, whether enzymes or any other agents, need to be conducted exclusively under the care of properly licensed physicians or medical professionals in strict accordance with the provisions of the law.

Many medical doctors have limited knowledge about enzymes or do not believe in their role for treatment. We also urge them to read this book as a re-introduction to a very exciting and highly important system within our bodies which may provide additional insight into their own modalities and philosophies of medical treatment. In this book, we simply present a review of medical information already published in respected international medical journals. A comprehensive bibliography is included and may be reviewed by the intcrested readers or their physicians.

Future of therapeutic enzymes

Despite the controversies, we feel that the therapeutic use of enzymes is likely to become a major form of medical treatment in the future. Their therapeutic potential is enormous! We believe that enzymes are the treatment of the future! Learning more about the pathophysiology of an illness and discovering associated enzyme defects can lead to replacement or addition of the required healthy enzyme, resulting in a treatment at the most basic and natural level. When better understood, enzymes may indeed represent some of the 'magic bullets' cited by Erlich.

Chapter 1

The "Fountain of Life"

Just imagine someone saying to you, "Your body contains countless millions of tiny building blocks, which continually renew, maintain and save your life. You would drop dead without them! Without them, you could not have been born. Not a single person, plant or animal would exist without them. They are the fountain of life. They are a magic force, the life energy, the labor force that keeps us alive. Mastering them will make us healthier and keep us alive longer. It can give us substantial control over our health and our lives."

If something like this exists, you ought to know about it. Everyone should know about it. It should be on everyone's lips. However, most people, in fact, have only a vague idea concerning these fantastic little building blocks which we call enzymes.

This common lack of knowledge about something so important to our bodies is actually very difficult to understand. An enormous amount is known about enzymes; they are one of the most important factors governing our lives and our health. And yet, despite the lack of interest and understanding about enzymes, according to new research, application of the overall knowledge and advances in this field make it possible to offer relief from some chronic diseases and possibly to prevent some illnesses.

We believe that this knowledge will eventually change our world as a whole with its applications in technology, industry, the environment and other fields.

Although not widelyknown in the United States or the Americas, the European research and experience has generated great excitement in the scientific community. The Europeans suggest that, "this knowledge can be used today to alleviate the pain which millions of people have had to suffer for years, and can be used preventively to protect us from new illnesses and to provide us with a longer, healthier life." In the United States, the average person generally does not know much about enzymes, their importance, what they actually are, or their power. Many persons have the wrong impressions or have been informed incorrectly. Many physicians also feel helpless due to lack of awareness or because of prejudices or 'prior medical dogma'. Indeed, the new European research appears to challenge this prevailing medical dogma. For these reasons, it is worthwhile for everyone to acquire some of this knowledge, and to understand some of the fascinating relationships which then become evident. This knowledge is certainly sufficient to help each of us personally to take better control of our health and place our fate into our own hands.

Enzymes are the accelerators of every single biochemical process. Are they indeed so important that they can justly be called the "Fountain of Life"?

If the world was created by Divine Power, one realizes that life on it was created through enzymes, the elemental energy source or basic life force. They were used to start, maintain and eventually end this life. It is only in the presence of enzymes that inanimate material can change, that controlled biochemical metabolism takes place and that vital energy becomes available. It was probably lightening and the ultraviolet light from the sun which provided the first impulses of energy for the formation of the building blocks of life, the so-called amino acids. Some of the amino acids combined to form enzymes. It was enzymes that then activated the other amino acids. Enzymes are responsible for synthesizing, joining together and duplicating whole chains of such amino acids and, thus, enabling the production of living organisms. These amino acid chains are known as proteins. Egg white, for instance, is largely protein. Enzymes themselves, are nothing different than proteins.

The history of life on earth to the present day can be comprehended by considering the enzymes required for evolution at each individual stage. Oxygen was produced in the air because particular new enzymes that set oxygen free were produced by simple plants. These plants had learned to produce certain enzymes which released oxygen from the carbon dioxide of the air and other substances. At present we know how this takes place. Enzymes which cause such reactions are now understood very well. Several scientists have been awarded the Nobel prize for solving this puzzle.

Do we copy Creation?

Scientists are already able to recreate some of these enzymes. The first successes were achieved in the investigation and imitation of photosynthesis. Scientists can use gene technology to influence bacteria to synthesize those enzymes which are required for the initiation of primitive life.

We can safely leave the discussion of whether this is "Creation" to moral theologists. Nonetheless, scientists have in this manner built a bridge between the calculable world of biological laws and the limitless regions of metaphysical omnipotence. The enzyme is to a biochemist what the soul is to a theologist.

We are, however, a long way from being able to breathe life into a robot and thus produce enchanting beauty queens or Frankenstein's monster as desired in the biochemical laboratory. So far, scientists have only mastered a few of the simplest enzymes. The most primeval cell owed its existence to the presence of such simple enzymes. As evolution progressed, more and different types of enzymes combined to form chains of interlinked reactions. Scientists believe that the living organisms which thereby developed became more varied and complex, and multiplied, leading eventually to the peak of Creation, the human being.

This leads to you, the reader. You are not the same person reading this sentence that you were when you picked this book up; during every second of your life, your more than 3,000 different enzymes, i.e. the number so far identified, together with their undiscovered colleagues, are in the process of performing, changing and renewing, sometimes at breath-taking speed, all that is necessary to keep you alive. They do all of this in an interlocking network which no computer can even begin to perform. During these last few seconds, millions of body cells have died off, been broken down and carried away, and millions of new ones have been produced as replacements. This is all taking place incidentally, as it were, merely a part of the innumerable range of tasks which have to be performed in order to keep us alive and healthy.

The reason why so many people fail to give enzymes the attention they deserve is based on ignorance and, to some extent, on prevailing, unsubstantiated dogma.

Perhaps the extensive variety, complexity and immense importance of enzymes threatens to overwhelm. Another reason may be the instinctive respect some people have, preventing them from delving into a region which they feel should remain out of limits; the feeling that an order they perceive as related to the origin of life, under Divine influence, should not to be subjected to manipulation and certainly not to imitation. These are the people who are concerned about science explaining aspects of creation. For example, we now know precisely which enzymes are responsible for keeping our blood in a steady state in order to help us to take in oxygen when we breathe and thus provide the cells with energy. We are learning more about which enzymes maintain our lives by many metabolic processes, and how. It will not be very long before scientists utilizing enzymes can recreate some of the most basic aspects of primitive life by means of genetic engineering. The knowledge obtained will be applied to improve our health, for the good of mankind.

There is no need to be terrified of this prospect. What use is it for us to be able to imitate the best of enzymes while still pondering the mystery of how the enzymes are able to communicate with each other, to harmonize and yet follow the instructions of an unknown higher control? If we never work out what natural laws govern the equilibrium between the completely different, simultaneously acting and reacting enzyme systems, how can we discover what higher principles control the pure chemical and physical mechanics?

It is not a question of competing with Divine creative powers. Science has not set itself the aim of learning the ways of all processes involving enzymes in order to create new life. The goal, rather, is to obtain an ever greater understanding of how life functions in order to be able to preserve it better and to once again make impaired life healthy.

Attaining and applying knowledge

Enzyme researchers active throughout the entire world have made astonishing strides along this path.

Naturally, there is still much knowledge to be learned which should eventually lead us to this goal. There are many unknown fields awaiting their discoverers. Whenever enzymes or enzyme therapy are mentioned, skeptics have an opportunity to say that it is not possible to make any reliable predictions about enzymes, or even about the treatment of disease with enzymes, since there is still so much that has not yet been proven scientifically. As in any field, advances in science cannot be expected to reach a point where no more new discoveries, or the changes which these entail, can be expected. Scientific research is an open-ended occupation.

Therefore, we cannot simply relax just because our understanding of the interactions between enzyme systems is increasing, because we are better able to reinforce these systems day-by-day in order to restore ourselves and maintain our health. We cannot say to those people who could be helped that they must wait since everything will be even better in the future. We must use this available knowledge and we must perfect our present abilities, so that we may be able to implement the opportunities now!

It is a matter of life and death. Our lives and our deaths. Enzymes play a role at the beginning and at the end of our existence and that is what this book is about.

Chapter 2

History: The "Magic Wand"

It could have been the Chinese who first noted this life force. In the same way that the ancient Chinese thousands of years ago gained so much knowledge from sources which are no longer accessible to us today, they might also have had an inkling of what energetic powers heaven, earth and all that lie between had led to; to the harmony of life.

There is absolutely no doubt, however, that the old world Egyptians, the Greeks and the Arabs later sensed that an unseen force existed which was responsible for changes in living organisms. A mysterious force which seemingly automatically changed one substance into another; milk into cheese, malt wort into beer, grape juice into wine or dough into bread.

The Ancient Egyptians searched for the magic wand to transform materials because they dreamed of the power and the wealth that would ensue from the possession of this knowledge. The Ancient Greeks on the other hand, believed that the Gods alone were capable of accomplishing such a wonder.

Only one Greek dared to try imitating this wonder. He patiently mixed many substances together in order to produce new ones in the process. One of the meanings of the Greek word *chymos* is juice. This Greek was Zosimos, 'the chymist'. In order to avoid prosecution for blasphemy on account of his activities, Zosimos moved to Egypt at the end of the 3rd century B.C. and attempted to unravel the secrets of nature with the best contemporary scientists there.

The Arabs referred to Zosimos' activity as *al kimiya* which is the origin of our term 'alchemy'. Zosimos referred to the divine power he sought as 'Xerion'. As far as the Arabs were concerned, *al kimiya* was a search for the philosopher's stone or magic potion, in Arabic *al iksir*. This name for the philosopher's stone has descended to us with the word 'elixir'. The medieval alchemists sought to find that omnipotent elixir in earth, metals, plants and animals. According to the dark mysteries of the Arabs, they were "in search of that all-healing force which could transmute sickness to health, death to life and base metals to eternal gold."

There were thousands of theories concerning this 'force'. No one disputed the existence of the 'unknown elixir', but there was no solid evidence as to where it was and how it might function.

The gizzard of the hawk

Then came Réaumur. He is only remembered today as the inventor of a temperature scale and, for a long time, temperatures were indeed measured in degrees Réaumur. However, this René Antoine Ferchant de Réaumur who lived from 1683 to 1757, principally in Paris, was one of the universal scientists who are hardly conceivable in today's age of specialization. He was a technologist, physicist and scientist. It was as an entomologist, in particular, that he enjoyed a reputation far beyond the boundaries of France.

During the last years of his life, Réaumur considered that the 'mysterious force' could best be sought where it was most readily discerned, namely in the transformation of food within the body, i.e. in digestion. In those days, it was still believed that food was ground mechanically in the stomach and then liquefied by the addition of gastric juice.

Réaumur had his doubts about this. He conferred with a young and promising colleague and friend, a very unusual priest from Pavia named Lazzaro Spallanzani. Réaumur's thoughts proceeded as follows: If a bird of prey is fed a small perforated metal capsule filled with a piece of meat and the bird then regurgitates the indigestible pellet, it can be seen whether the meat in the capsule remains unaffected because it could not be broken down mechanically into small pieces or whether it would be digested by the postulated forces assumed in the stomach.

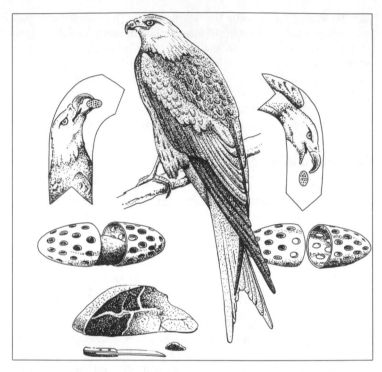

Figure 7:   The piece of meat within a perforated metal capsule is digested in the bird of prey's stomach

Réaumur carried out the first experiments along these lines and saw that the meat had actually disappeared from the regurgitated capsule, indicating the gizzard did not break up the food mechanically as had long been supposed (Figure 7).

Lazzaro Spallanzani liked this experiment. The Jesuit and biologist was particularly fond of unusual experiments, especially when they contradicted the biblical point of view. He had demonstrated the power of regeneration in brilliant experiments on the ability of lizards to regrow lost tails. According to published reports, he was the first person to carry out experiments of artificial insemination (with dogs) which, in itself, was somewhat outside the normal activities of a priest, even for a Jesuit.

However, it took about 30 years before Spallanzani paid closer attention to Réaumur's experiments. In 1783, he went to a falconry and arranged for meat-filled, perforated metal capsules to be fed to falcons and buzzards. As Réaumur had previously observed, the capsules were again empty after regurgitation.

This did not satisfy Spallanzani. He went further. He concluded that 'the force' altering the food must be contained in the gastric juice. This time, he filled the same metal capsules with a small sponge which soaked up gastric juice while inside the bird of prey. He then placed the gastric juice in a vessel with pieces of meat which, to Spallanzani's delight, were subsequently dissolved. For the first time, it was thereby clear that gastric juice contains a substance which dissolves proteins. These results became well-known in an astonishingly short period of time. Only two years after the experiment was performed, a German book was published in Leipzig with the imposing title, "The Abbot Spallanzani's Experiments on the Digestion of Humans and Various Animal Species, with Remarks by Mr. Senebier."

The remarks of Jean Senebier in the appendix of this book should not be ignored. Jean Senebier (1742–1809) was a young friend of Spallanzani. He was another exceptionally talented and inventive scientist, another man of the church, minister of ecclesiastical affairs of the Canton of Geneva, Switzerland. Senebier had immediately drawn his own conclusions from Spallanzani's experiments and applied animal gastric juice to the poorly healing wounds and open varicose ulcers of several patients, with success. The proliferative, inflamed tissue was dissolved and healing could begin. Senebier was not the first to use 'proteolytic' (protein-dissolving) enzymes in medicine. It had been done since the dawn of time, generally with plant poultices, but he was probably the first enzyme therapist who had at least some idea of what he was actually doing.

The discovery of enzymes

Naturally, scientists wanted to find out what was 'the force' in the gastric juice that brought about this dissolution. Gastric juice was also found to contain hydrochloric acid, leading to the solid scientific belief for half a century that this hydrochloric acid in the gastric juice was responsible for decomposing the proteins and making them available for the body's use. This continued to be maintained, even though experiments on the subject failed to confirm it, because scholars were not too particular in scrutinizing their opinions.

It was 1836, almost one-hundred years after the first experiments of Réaumur, before the physician and biochemist Theodor Schwann, whom we thank for the first knowledge concerning cellular structure and metabolism, and for understanding the nerve cells which bear his name, studied this 'digestive force'. He was able to isolate and concentrate a substance from gastric juice which was able to decompose and dissolve protein particularly readily. He named this substance *pepsin*.

Pepsin is evidently one of those substances sought from ancient times whose 'hidden force' or energy, in a mysterious way, leads to changes in proteins, the basic building blocks of all life. In those days, these substances did not yet have a name.

One could only speculate as to how such substances functioned. The Swedish scientist Jöns Jacob, Baron von Berzelius, was a man who, based on theoretical grounds, came to the correct hypothesis of this mechanism of action. In the same year that Schwann described *pepsin*, he published an article in which he wrote, "We have grounds for assuming that there are thousands of *catalytic processes* taking place between tissues and fluids in living plants and animals, and that they bring about varying amounts of degradation which we will probably discover in the catalytic powers of the organic tissue making up the organs of the body."

Catalysts! That was the answer to the mystery of the hidden force. Properly speaking, biocatalysts. These are particular substances whose presence effects and accelerates changes in an organic substance. Many forces that bring about changes outside human cells, alcohol fermentation for example, are also brought about by biocatalysts. Incidentally, this had already been postulated by Schwann.

The difference between biocatalysts active within and outside living cells was a topic which concerned Louis Pasteur. It was he who first used the term 'ferment' for the biocatalyst responsible for fermentation. However, the term was soon limited to those ferments reacting within the living cell.

It was the German natural philosopher, physician and professor of physiology Willy Kühne who, in 1878 in Heidelberg, introduced the word 'enzyme' for a biocatalyst that also altered protein outside the living cell. Thus, the term is not much older than one-hundred years.

The confusion which then followed between 'ferments' and 'enzymes' was ended officially in 1897 when it was stipulated that the term 'enzyme' should be used to refer to all biocatalysts. This, however, has not helped very much. The two terms are frequently used together or even interchangeably today. Let us forget the word 'ferment' and stick with 'enzyme'.

The time has now come to at least indicate what unbelievably fascinating and versatile substances enzymes are. It is time to unveil the magic wand of life which has continued to remain obscure.

Chapter 3

Biochemistry: The solution to the mystery

Scientists have discovered the composition of enzymes and how they function. There are numerous scientific publications on the nature of enzymes just awaiting your attention. Biochemists can justly point out that they have made tremendous strides in recent years toward understanding enzymatic processes.

We can therefore easily maintain that a good portion of the mystery has been solved, although it must be admitted that what is really meant is that some of the mysteries have been solved. However, an immeasurable number of other mysteries must still be unraveled before we actually hold the magic wand in our hands.

The explanations of the nature of enzymes offered in this chapter simply represent the ABC's of biochemistry. The reader will be thankful for this, since further penetration into the material would indeed be very impressive and fascinating, but it would also be confusing and fatiguing for the casual reader.

Presence suffices

Let us start quite simply with the concept of a 'catalyst'. You know about the catalyzer in the catalytic converter which we hope is attached to your new car. Its purpose is to exploit the heat of the exhaust gases and to convert toxic carbon monoxide into the less dangerous carbon dioxide. The catalyst does this merely by being present and is not altered in any manner in the process. The catalyst itself is not affected, it does not require any energy of its own.

If you wanted to convert carbon monoxide to carbon dioxide without a catalyst you would need to build an apparatus into the car which was as big as the car's motor and which would require more energy than the car engine itself.

Nature never wastes expense and energy, it always chooses the most economical route and is better than all the engineers in the world at this game. The trick with the catalyst is one of nature's favorites. Small causes, big effects!

Another example, a passionate young man suddenly confronted with a snapshot of his loved one is changed by this photo; his cheeks blush, his pulse quickens, he breathes heavily and other physical reactions may also occur. All this merely in the presence of a catalyst, the photo, which is not affected by any of this and remains unchanged.

Let us now choose a more appropriate example related to chemistry so that we can be taken more seriously. Take a lump of sugar and hold a burning match to it, the sugar will not burn. Now flick some ash onto the lump (perhaps a smoker carelessly left ash nearby) and apply the flame to the sugar again – it now burns. The ash contains the catalyst for combustion, i.e. the substance necessary for mediating the biochemical reaction (Figure 8).

Both inorganic and organic catalysts exist. Here, we are only concerned with the organic ones, the enzymes. These, in a dry, technological nutshell, are biocatalytically-active proteins with a high molecular mass and a complex structure.

Even if this sounds like part of a furthering education lesson, please be patient for a few more pages while some of the basic properties of these enzymes are described. The reader will surely find this worthwhile since he or she will then have a far greater understanding of what goes on in his or her body, why he or she is healthy or why he or she may be ill, and how enzymes can make the body healthy again.

How they are produced, how they function

It has been known for more than one-hundred years that enzymes are proteins. It has also been known for a long time that proteins consist of a chain of amino acids. However, it was not until 1959 when it became possible, as a result of the refinement

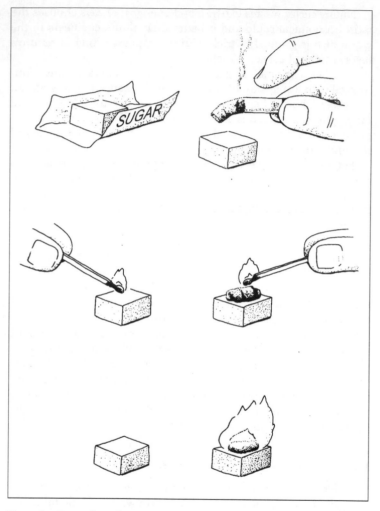

Figure 8:   Sugar alone does not burn (left), cigarette ash contains the catalyzer required for combustion (right)

in analytical techniques, to say how many amino acids are present in a given enzyme.

A number of amino acids become interconnected in specific 'amino acid chains' and, together, these chains become arranged to form the various polypeptides and proteins of the body. Each enzyme is composed of a very specific set of amino acid chains (Figure 9). There are 20 basic amino acids. At this point, we do not need to bother ourselves with their names.

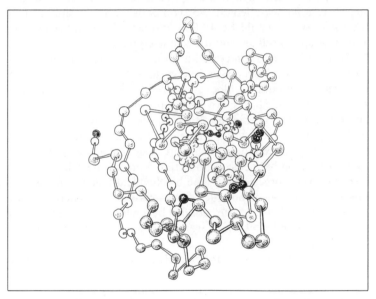

Figure 9: Enzyme molecule: The long 'string of pearls' made up of a contiguous amino acid chain is wound together like a ball of yarn (the darkly shaded portions signify active sites of the molecule)

All enzymes merely differ in the number and sequence of these 20 amino acids which are assembled into chains of varying lengths. For this reason, they all differ from each other a little in appearance. In general, you can picture any enzyme as follows; the amino acids are arranged like a string of pearls which is wound together like a ball of yarn in such a manner that there is an indentation at one point, a very precisely shaped opening. This opening is the focus of everything, it is the *active site* (Figure 9).

Enzymes are fairly large molecules, at least from a biochemist's viewpoint. Just one example for size, if the enzyme *trypsin*, one of the first enzymes to be investigated at the start of enzymological science, were magnified to be ten centimeters in size, it would stretch to a fantastic length. For comparison, a man enlarged to the same extent would be 40,000 kilometers tall and would be able to wrap himself around the whole equator.

Every living organism contains an unimaginable variety of different biochemical structures known as *substrates*. They are the raw material or building blocks required to build or repair our tissues or cells. Substrates are components necessary for one or another of life's processes and they flit about ready to be used. In so doing, they come near an enzyme and are attracted to its active site – if they fit exactly into this precisely shaped site, and only then, something happens; for one tiny moment the substrate and enzyme form a precise *unit*. The biochemical reaction for which this enzyme has been constructed then takes place. When the substrate is large in size, it is surrounded by a whole series of enzymes which alter it bit by bit. They are biochemical factories with enzymatic conveyor-belt activity.

Most enzyme activities involve cleavage of a substrate. Only about 3 to 5% of enzymes combine substrates, synthesizing instead of cleaving. These are the 'anabolic' enzymes and not the cleaving (catabolic) enzymes. When cleavage takes place, the substrate which fits into the active site is broken down and the pieces are then released in two portions. These are the two products of the reaction. One product may be regarded as waste and is used to produce new substrates after it has been broken down into its remaining biochemical components. The other product is a new substrate which can now search for a different enzyme to undergo another change. This process continues until a product is finally produced that has a particular function within the organism. The process resembles an assembly line for the step-by-step manufacture of parts and components which are then put together to finally build an automobile.

Lock and key

As can be seen, an enzyme is not a universal genius but a rather one-sided specialist. A biochemist would say that each enzyme is substrate-specific, or almost. There are exceptions to every rule, but, all in all, it is not very far from the truth to say that each enzyme type is only able to take up and alter one specific species of substrate in its precisely shaped active site.

Each enzyme is also reaction-specific. This means that it can only carry out one quite specific change on the substrate, producing one single effect.

One of the early biochemists, Professor Fischer, illustrated this beautifully with the example of a lock and key. It is only possible to unlock the lock when the wards of the key fit exactly into the keyhole. The enzyme is a lock with a very specific keyhole, the substrate is the key (Figure 10). In addition, the unlocking process can only be carried out in one particular way; similary, the key must either be turned to the left or right so that a bolt can open or a faucet can be turned on and off. Likewise, the enzymes produce one specific action in order that some other useful function can occur.

The logical question which now has to be faced is, "Since there are so many different substrates and so many different reactions all requiring their own specific enzymes, how many different types of enzymes do our bodies require?"

This is a question to which enzyme researchers are still addressing themselves. Only one enzyme was known in 1831. In 1930, the number had risen to a total of 80. By 1984, approximately 2,500 enzymes had been classified, subclassified and sub-

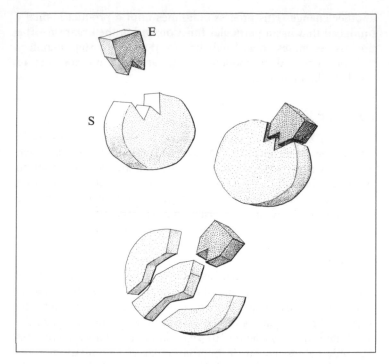

Figure 10: Substrates (S) fit precisely into the active site of an enzyme (E), like a key
            in a lock. The substrate is cleaved subsequently and the enzyme remains
            unchanged

subclassified. In 1993, approximately 3,000 enzymes are recognized. The end of the search is nowhere in sight, even though some scientists think they see light at the end of the tunnel. Some surprises are still entirely possible. Is the number ten thousand? Is it even larger? Will we ever recognize all the enzymes?

There are, at least as the prestigious Enzyme Commission of the International Union of Biochemistry has finally stated, six groups of enzymes with 6 fundamentally different enzymatic activities. One group, for instance, is concerned with the transport of electrons from a donor to an acceptor which, aside from other actions, is of vital importance for cell respiration. Another group transfers a whole molecule from a donor to an acceptor, i.e. it moves fragments from one part of an amino acid chain to another. Yet another group changes the substrate by rearranging a certain molecular group of the substrate. A further group provides energy for other biosynthetic processes by catalyzing the cleavage of energy-rich substrates. The fifth group breaks up each substrate molecule into two parts and the final group is able to cleave compounds into smaller parts. Since the enzymes in this last group perform cleavage by introducing a molecule of water, they are known as *hydrolases*. When a biochemical substance is given a name ending in '...*ase*', you can be pretty certain that it is one of the 3,000 or so enzymes which exist. The names given at the very beginning of enzyme research were different, they usually ended in '...*in*' as with *pepsin* and *trypsin* which have already been discussed. They were among the first enzymes to be studied more intensively.

The group of hydrolytic enzymes will be especially emphasized in this book since they are of particular importance. They are enzymes we already know a great deal about. They can help us to re-establish and protect our health.

All 3,000 or more different enzymes are constantly being produced en masse by our body. That is a fantastic performance, but there is one small drawback; some of these enzymes lack a small portion to perfect the shape making up the active site, so that the substrate would simply escape again from the hole making up the reaction site. A complementary piece, known as a *coenzyme*, is required to complete the fit of the active site. In order to produce the coenzyme needed to complete the template of the active site (Figure 11), we have to consume the materials essential for its construction, since our bodies, unfortunately, are incapable of making the coenzymes from the available components.

A piece of the jigsaw puzzle is missing

We have to ingest the material for constructing the coenzyme in our food. Even when the quantities involved are sometimes tiny, certain enzymes cannot be manufactured in the absence of a coenzyme. Furthermore, without these particular enzymes (functionally complete with their coenzymes), the whole enzymatic system falls out of equilibrium and we become ill. If the materials required are unavailable for a longer period of time, we may even die (Figure 11).

Everyone is surely familiar with the components required for producing these coenzymes. They include vitamins, trace elements and minerals. Everybody is probably also aware that these are essential for life.

Not every vitamin is essential only because it is needed for the production of a coenzyme. This is principally the function of vitamins B_1, B_2, B_6, B_{12} and vitamins C and K, together with some less well-known vitamins.

The husk of the rice grain is one good source of vitamin B_1. Anyone who lives almost exclusively from polished rice will be deficient in vitamin B_1 and suffer the almost classical avitaminosis 'beriberi'. This, incidentally, is a Singhalese word meaning 'great weakness'. Vitamin B_{12} deficiency leads to a blood condition known as pernicious anemia. Or consider the seafarers of earlier days who were deprived of fresh vegetables and fruit for months at a time and came down with scurvy as a result of vitamin C deficiency.

In fact, every disturbance of enzyme equilibrium results in illness. A vitamin deficiency or a lack of other substances needed to produce coenzymes can cause disturbances in the body which result in specific illnesses.This happens in cases of trace elements and mineral deficiencies. These materials include both metals and minerals; copper and iron, nickel, manganese, molybdenum, selenium, the important element magnesium, as well as sodium,, potassium and zinc. The trace element zinc alone is an essential component of coenzymes required for the proper function of 80 different enzymes.

These coenzymes are something quite different from enzymes. Enzymes are composed of protein whereas the coenzymes are not. Enzymes are enormous, while coenzymes are very small molecules. Enzymes are not degraded during their activities whereas coenzymes are and therefore require continual regeneration or renewal.

However, all this has again taken us far too far into the biochemical jungle. Let us leave it at that. There is, however, quite another interesting story to be told about coenzymes. Some substances are almost identical with such coenzyme components. Let's call them pseudo-coenzymes. They are so similar that they can be mistaken for the actual coenzymes and the body occasionally makes a mistake and lets these similar substances fit into the active site of the enzyme. The completed enzyme is therefore unable to perform its task and we become ill as a result of this built-in error.

It is quite simple to poison rats in this way. A frequently employed rat and mouse poison contains the vegetable aroma warfarin. Warfarin is readily mistaken by the human and animal body for the coenzyme vitamin K, which plays a decisive role in the production of enzymes essential for blood coagulation. Thus, if the body is provided with warfarin, it incorporates it into the enzymes in place of vitamin K, meaning that several enzymes essential for blood clotting can no longer function. The blood is liquefied to such an extent that the rats and mice die of internal bleeding.

That is a bad thing for the rats and mice, but a good thing for some patients who suffer from blood which is 'too thick', since they can be treated orally or by injection with medicaments containing small quantities of warfarin (coumarin), and the sticky blood becomes more liquid.

It is astonishing how it is already possible to control the activities of enzymes and deliberately employ them as needed since scientists have found out what they look like and what working conditions they like. They are, indeed, very dependent on certain specific conditions.

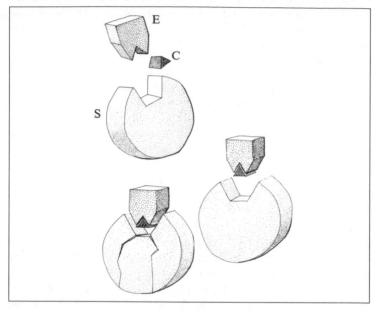

Figure 11: The substrate (S) only fits into the active site of the enzyme (E) after its template has been altered by a coenzyme (C).

Best working conditions are mandatory

The question as to whether the beneficial effects enzymes bring about by their mere presence can be referred to as 'work' is best left to the sociologist.

At any rate, enzymes make some demands on their environments for their well-being and optimal action. They are, for instance, temperature-dependent. The enzymes active in the human body develop their highest activity at around body temperature, with activity increasing as the temperature rises to that of a high fever. At about 40 °C (104 °F) the enzymes are in a 'fever' of activity. For this reason, our bodies raise the temperature when a crisis occurs, naturally with the aid of enzymes, and the fever enhances the activity of the enzymes desperately needed to combat that crisis. The body does this unwillingly and only in cases of emergency. Indeed, if the temperature is raised just a little more and the optimal peak temperature is exceeded by just a small amount, the whole system of enzyme activity collapses. The protein of the enzymes coagulates, solidifies and loses its functional abilities. In this way, the person dies. On the other hand, enzyme activity slows down as the temperature is decreased. This is why butter and cheese stay fresh in the refrigerator. The reduced enzyme activity makes life in the butter and cheese go on much more slowly.

When surgeons intend to sew a finger or toe back on, it is essential that they cool the separated appendage, as cool as say champagne, for transport to the hospital. Freezing, however, is not tolerated well. Storage should not be below 0 °C (32 °F). The same applies to the transport of livers, kidneys and other organs for transplantation.

We can now take the opportunity of answering the question which is so important in our clock and speedometer-dominated age; how fast are enzymes? How long do they need to attract a substrate to their active sites, to alter it and to release it once again? The answer is once again typical for enzymology, 'it depends'.

Each enzyme develops its own working speed which is adapted to the particular working conditions. We can, however, get some idea of the sort of speed at which an enzyme works by considering the slowest enzyme that we know, *lysozyme* (its purpose, for example, is to help in the destruction of bacteria); it is able to process about 30 substrate molecules per minute. That is all of 2 seconds for each molecule. This contrasts with the fastest worker of all, namely carbonic anhydrase (you can immediately forget the name); it processes a fantastic 36 million substrate molecules in one minute.

Before your admiration for carbonic anhydrase passes all bounds and your contempt for lysozyme becomes too great, you should realize that the speed of substrate transformation is not the same thing as the intensity of action. An explanation of why this is so would involve a laborious journey through the biochemical jungle. It naturally has to do with the working conditions.

A further ideal working condition demanded by enzymes is the correct surroundings. Each enzyme type feels good in particular surroundings. They require an environment which is either somewhat on the acidic side or slightly basic. The biochemist would say, "Every enzyme has an optimal pH."

In addition, an enzyme's 'desire' to work is dependent on whether there is a large amount of substrate waiting to be changed or whether a great deal of product has already been built up. The more substrate, the higher the activity of the enzyme. The more substrate breakdown product present, the lower the enzyme activity.

Living and dying for the common good

As has already been mentioned several times, the activity of an enzyme is not activity in the usual sense, it is merely the presence of an unaltered protein body which brings about a particular effect. However, this statement is not one-hundred percent true either.

Every protein alters with time and does not exist eternally. They age, meaning that enzymes age as well. Their state of perfection continues to deteriorate and eventually the active site ceases to be a true template, errors occur. When an enzyme begins to exhibit such signs of wear, i.e. when it is overaged, another enzyme comes along and makes short work of it. The colleague-in-arms is degraded, dissolved and transported away without so much as a good-bye. This cannibalism functions because enzymes have a preference for denatured protein, or in other words, sick tissue. When a colleague-in-arms is denatured it is just a special tidbit.

Some enzymes only have a life-span of about 20 minutes and then must be replaced by a newly produced enzyme of the same type. Others remain active for several weeks before they have to be replaced because of their age.

The fact that some enzymes consume other enzymes should not be thought of in terms of enmity. On the contrary, one of the most fascinating properties of all enzymes is their ability to work with each other, to form themselves into cooperatives if necessary, and to continually exchange information with other enzyme cooperatives. In this way, they maintain a common effort with a joint goal resulting in the equilibrium of all systems and harmony within all processes of life.

This cannot be brought about by any single enzyme alone. Each enzyme cannot just function for itself with the hope that everything will be all right. The comprehension of this cooperative function of all enzymes for the common good and in the absence of a dictator might inspire us to be able to develop the ideal form of government. Enzymes often work consecutively in steps one after another, in so-called enzyme cascades, in order to perform important, complex tasks within the body and thus maintain the system in an ideal state between excess and deficiency (Figure 12).

One enzyme activates the next enzyme which then activates a further enzyme and then another and another, until a last enzyme finally triggers the desired effect. One of the reasons for this method is economy, since such small steps require far less energy than one larger, more complex step. Safety is another reason. Blood coagulation and liquefication are examples. So are the contraction and dilatation of the blood vessels, and the triggering and

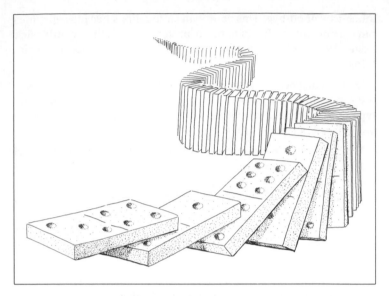

Figure 12: Enzyme cascade: As with a row of falling dominoes, one enzyme activates the next enzyme which then activates a further enzyme and so forth
until a last enzyme finally triggers the desired effect

activation of the forces of defense, such as seen in the immune
system.

For the body, it is essential that these activities remain on the
narrow course between excess and deficiency and not become too
extreme. Otherwise we would suffer from arteriosclerosis or be in
danger of becoming hemophiliacs, we would suffer from hyper-
tension or even hypotension, or if our resistance did not function
properly, we would die from the next attack of germs or other
pathogens.

Keeping on the safe side

These risks are present because enzymes are stubborn specialists, carrying out their functions without delay. Whether the substrate presented comes from the human body, or is animal or vegetable in origin, is all the same to them. If the shape of the substrate fits the template of the active site and the general working conditions are in order, the enzyme will cause its specific effect no matter what. This fact is responsible for the versatility of enzymes, but it can also be dangerous if they work away with uncontrolled activity. For this reason, every living organism is not only equipped with the mandatory enzymes, but also with a double safety system to prevent these enzymes from coming into action unintentionally.

This is understandable. A question that is posed time and again is, "Why don't protein-degrading enzymes simply break us down, since we are principally made up of proteins?" Or consider the case of *pepsin* which breaks down the proteins of the food in the stomach. Why does it not break down the stomach itself which is also made of protein?

The double safety system works, again simplified, as follows: The enzymes which are continually replaced in our bodies, are not initially active. There are special amino acids in a position on the amino acid chains which block their activity, just like the *safety catch* on a Colt.

These harmless enzymes swim throughout the blood and lymph streams, millions of completely innocuous structures. Only when a particular enzyme reaction is required at some point in the body does another, in the same way a separate, specially activated enzyme, release the safety catch. The enzyme is only now ready and able to change any substrate it meets. This is the first safety system.

Enzyme inhibitors make up the second safety system (Figure 13). These enzyme inhibitors produced endogenously (within the organism) are able to occupy the active sites of enzymes and thus put these out of action when too much active enzyme is present. Some enzyme inhibitors remain attached to the enzyme for the remainder of its life, others detach themselves again so that the temporarily inhibited enzyme can once more become active.

Exogenous enzyme inhibitors (produced outside of the organism) are also known. The rat poison warfarin already mentioned is an example. Indeed, many poisons act in this way. Snake and insect venoms function via enzyme inhibitors which knock out certain enzymes of the organism affected. They bring the metabolism out of equilibrium to such an extent that the organism may die if the enzymes which fail are not replaced in time.

Numerous other substances have been discovered which can be used to neutralize quite specific enzymes and thus deliberately interfere with the metabolic processes. Many drugs function this way. The world's best-known drug functions according to this principle. It was a long time before this was realized and *aspirin* had been administered in inconceivable quantities for decades without the reason for its effects being known.

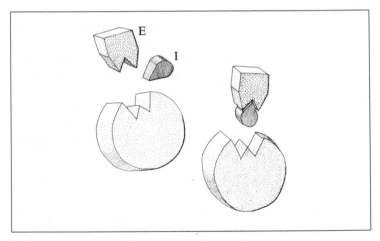

Figure 13: An enzyme inhibitor (I) blocks the active site of an enzyme (E)

Aspirin consists of acetylsalicylic acid. This acid is an exogenous substance which can attach itself to an enzyme that plays a role in coagulation and in inflammatory processes. This enzyme has the complicated name *cyclooxygenase*. In this way, the acid inhibits coagulation and the blood therefore becomes thinner. Its inhibition of the inflammatory process leads to reduced inflammation and reduced pain.

Consider antibiotics like penicillin or steroids such as cortisone as well. The ultimate mechanism of action results in a willful disturbance of the activity of a particular enzyme as a result of attachment of the inhibitor to the active site.

These are only a few examples of the exploitation of our knowledge concerning enzymes. A knowledge which we can only just touch on here if we do not wish to try the patience of our readers.

However, patience pays off. If you have actually read this chapter attentively, you belong to a small but select number of individuals who have learned some fundamental concepts about a subject that is decisive to our health, our recovery from illness and our life as a whole.

Chapter 4

Nature and technology: The genie from the bottle

Legends, the ancient legends at least, are full of meaning and symbolic power. Like the fairy tale from 'Tales of the Thousand and One Nights', the story of the young man who finds a bottle in the shallow water of a beach; he opens it and a wisp arises from the bottle taking the form of a genie who can fulfill every wish. This legend is closely bound with the alchemy of the Arabs. It is reminiscent of the attempts by the medieval alchemists to conjure up the spirit of the true elixir from their glass vessels. It is also associated with the only force that mankind had bottled over thousands of years and which is able to perform many wonders; the force that converts the sweet juice of the grape into wine.

It is believed that such a force must be hidden wherever life is present. Only a question of bringing it out of hiding and turning it into a willing slave to fulfill all wishes remains. How will the dream of taming the omnipotent enzyme become reality?

There is no point in enumerating where enzymes are hidden in nature. Enzymes can be found everywhere, in people, animals, plants, foods, and in the tiny microorganisms which make up the boundary between living and nonliving matter. Here, we provide only a few examples of how nature exploits enzymes and the purposes for which they are applied, in addition to their use in the production and reproduction of life.

Enzymes in nature since Adam and Eve

Had his mind not been elsewhere, Adam might have observed an example of such enzymatic activity after having bitten into the fruit offered to him by Eve. Let's assume, as many theologians believe, that the fruit was an apple. The surface of the apple where the bite had been taken became coated with an ever browner layer (Figure 14). This process which is set in action by enzymes is the apple's immediate attempt to close this large wound. It is a protective layer intended to prevent the inside of the apple from drying out and being attacked by bacteria, molds and other dangers. At the same time, a healing process is set in motion by other enzymes just under the protective surface, to preserve the rest of the apple.

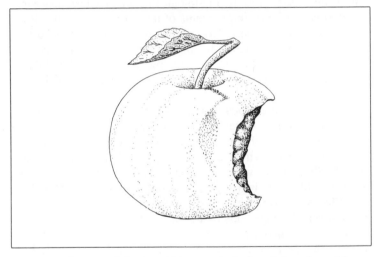

Figure 14: When an apple has been bitten, a protective layer is formed over this area with the help of enzymes

When you are injured, you too begin immediately to form a protective layer with the aid of alarmed and activated enzymes based on the same principles.

Nature has many ways of protecting itself from hostile influences and the attacks of enemies, ways that involve refined systems of enzymes.

Mushrooms demonstrate no physical protection. They have no thorns, nor hard shell, some of them therefore try to protect themselves from being eaten by being poisonous, forming a poison which causes enzymatic damage in anything that eats them. The human organism has no enzymes capable of capturing these mycotoxins, degrading and eliminating them.

However, over the course of evolution, some animals have learned to develop such enzymes. Pigs, for instance, otherwise astonishingly similar to us physiologically, do have enzymes capable of breaking down the proteins of mycotoxins. Humans, however, lack these enzymes. This special enzyme is synthesized by a bacterium in the stomach of the pig. Many animals exist which are insensitive to snake bites or insect stings which would be fatal in other species and this all on account of the enzymes which are present.

There is also a curious example of this enzymatic warfare in the plant kingdom. A plant grows in Africa with an appearance very similar to that of our forget-me-not (bluebird or myositis). It is a tremendously sensitive, delicate plant, but requires a large area to flourish as well. The vigorously growing neighboring plants would normally overgrow it and it would perish. Therefore, it produces a toxin containing fluorine which is washed to the roots of neighboring plants by the rain. The neighboring plants do not possess an enzyme able to decompose this toxin so that they all die. That is, all except for an insignificant looking little herb which has developed the necessary enzyme and can thus survive. After a long period of rain, the site is inhabited by practically only the sensitive, poison-producing 'killer plant' and the little, inconspicuous herb with its enzymatic antidote.

An unusual story, but nature even provides more remarkable phenomena. Enzymes are capable of producing light without any additional energy requirement – cold light. Every glowworm can do this as well. The phenomenon is known as bioluminescence, a term which means something like 'living light'. Not only glowworms and their blinking relatives in many tropical countries flash their living lights, many fish, crustaceans and sponges in the dark depths of the oceans are also bioluminescent, as are some beetles, millipedes and worms. The so-called railroad worm of Uruguay is a particularly interesting example. It can even glow in two colors. Along the right and left sides of its body are rows of little green 'lamps', and in the front, on its head, it has two red 'lamps'. It alone knows why.

We have no need to go diving into the depths of the ocean or to far away Uruguay in our search for a further living thing capable of bioluminescence; we ourselves perform the feat, albeit rather weakly. Macrophages, important phagocytic cells in our immune systems, can also glow. Our intestines can glow as well. The latter is performed by exogenic microorganisms possessing the enzymes which function specifically for this purpose.

Enzymes do not seem to have any limits. Nature has learned to pack these essential, temperature-sensitive enzymes in the embryo of one species of shrimp in such a way that the embryos can survive virtually forever in the arid desert or in the eternal ice. Microorganisms have been discovered whose enzymes feel at home in volcanic lava at 100 °C and which die off when the lava no longer boils. Thus, there is life in volcanic lava. There is also life in sulfur. Sulfur bacteria can feed on sulfur enzymatically. There are tiny bacteria that enzymatically alter the iron in some iron mines. Here, the dream of bringing metals to life approaches reality.

The alchemists had a premonition of what the genie in the bottle could do. Science is gradually providing the explanation.

Technology follows nature

Understandably, the more scientists learned about the world of enzymes, the more they wished to tempt this wonderful genie out of its bottle and put it to use.

The field in which scientists are trying to achieve this is biotechnology. It has thus far developed in four stages:

1. *Prescientific Era.* From the dawn of mankind to about 1800, some biological processes were exploited with scarcely an idea of the mechanism behind them.
2. *Early Scientific Era.* The time from 1800 to 1900, a period during which the first important principles of biochemistry were discovered and during which a start was made on the conscious exploitation of the biological transformation of materials.
3. *Biotechnology Era.* The time after 1900 when industry recognized the limitless possibilities of biotechnology which they developed and employed on an ever larger scale.
4. *Genetic Engineering Era.* The time since 1970 with the beginning of genetic engineering and thereby the start of an age where it appears possible to train and tame enzymes.

The Bible already provides numerous examples of biotechnology. Namely, it deals with the conversion of grapes to wine, of dough to bread and of milk to cheese. Anyone who sits down to have a glass of wine, a slice of bread and a piece of cheese is partaking of the longest-known products of deliberately applied biotechnology. These are the foundations on which the modern biotechnological industry has based the present-day standards. Better understanding of enzymes thus obtained is essential for our health, and to improve our daily life and certainly our survival on earth. Modern rescue from environmental catastrophes has also benefited immensely from the application of genetic engineering-controlled enzyme technology.

Industrial biotechnology – common uses of enzymes: Beer, bread, chocolate, mayonnaise

Let us stay with the simpler examples of biotechnology. The greatest quantities of enzymes are probably used by beer brewers.

Thousands of tons of the *amylases* bound to the malt ensure fermentation. Amylases are digestive enzymes such as those also produced in our bodies. They are concerned with the conversion of starch into sugars, with fermentation, and they are nowadays controlled in the breweries by means of ever more complicated and refined biotechnological processes.

It is also the amylase in the yeast which converts dough to bread. Amylase, a word which is derived from the Greek and means 'in sourdough', is, thus, the original 'enzyme'. Originally this indicated 'the substance in yeast that brings about the change' and was, as we now know, *amylase*.

Starch is decomposed by amylase, a process that is absolutely essential for the food industry. The earlier sources of amylase were *malt, cereal grains and also such microorganisms as molds*. Chocolate syrup, for instance, is manufactured by decomposing cocoa starch with amylases obtained from various plants.

Nowadays, the manufacture of most amylases has become routine. The biotechnological industry can virtually supply to order. Industrial biotechnological needs are enormous and not limited to amylases alone, but include an almost indescribable variety of other enzymes. They are required for the preservation of many foods, such as in increasing the shelf-life of mayonnaise, milk powder or cornflakes, for manufacturing sweeteners, clarifying fruit juices and for thousands of other things.

The tenderizer

The meat industry relies on enzymes to make meat tender. The famous experiments by Réaumur and Spallanzani made it clear that enzymes break down the protein of meat. It is also known why meat gets tender when it is 'hung' in cold storage. At this temperature, the protein-cleaving enzymes, the *proteases*, function with reduced activity. The meat can thus be controlled so that it becomes tender slowly. It can therefore be served at the right stage of degradation before it has become unpalatable by further degradation. At higher temperatures, the activities of the proteases would be supported to such an extent that the meat would rapidly decay and even liquefy. Additionally, it would be exposed to bacterial attack.

All a matter of cheese

If we are to believe one ancient legend, the discovery of cheese is attributed to a stroke of fate which befell an Arabian merchant. Allah be praised! This merchant travelled aimlessly and unsuspectingly through the desert with his camel, taking milk with him for his refreshment which he kept in a pouch made from a sheep's stomach and hung to the side of his camel (Figure 15). The warmth of the sun, motion of the camel and the digestive enzyme still present in the sheep's stomach transformed the milk to soft cheese and whey as the merchant travelled. The Arabian merchant was thus provided with both food and drink, and became the father of cheese.

It soon became clear that the digestive enzyme found in the sheep's stomach was the actual starter for cheese production. It is today called *chymosin* or *rennin* in biotechnology. It was actually the first enzyme that could be isolated.

Rennin has been used for cheese production for hundreds of years. It is obtained from the fourth stomach of all ruminants, although only from the very young ones, the calves and lambs. However, the digestive enzyme *pepsin* appears in that part of their stomach together with chymosin as soon as calves and lambs start to eat grass, and this cannot be used for cheese production since, among other things, it alters the taste. Incidentally, babies also have rennin in their stomachs initially before it disappears from their digestive system as their diet becomes diversified. If a baby that has only been fed milk spits some of this out, it smells cheesy as a result of this rennin.

Previously, there was sufficient rennin available from calf stomachs. However, as meat production increased, the numbers of

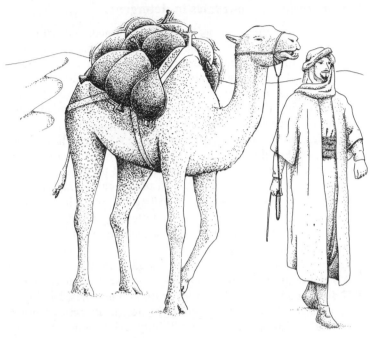

Figure 15: The "discovery" of cheese

young dairy calves being slaughtered began to fall and, together with the increased cheese production, raised the demand for rennin.

A search was therefore made for substitute enzymes, none of which has proven to be as well-suited as rennin. Incidentally, Italian cheeses are often started with an enzyme obtained from the jugular glands of calves and lambs, a peculiarity which is responsible for the spicy flavor of many Italian cheeses.

The biotechnological industry has since solved the problem of rennin. It is now produced by specially trained strains of cheap and willing microorganisms.

A clean business – enzymes in detergents

The proteases and amylases already mentioned, with which so much has been achieved in the food industry, have also been exploited by the detergent industry for the manufacture of washing powders. However, a small problem here was that the proteases obtained from animal sources were able to dissolve particles of dirt, although they were not suitable for boiled wash since the enzymes were destroyed at high temperatures.

The first enzymatic detergent was not, as might have been expected, marketed in the United States, but in Holland in 1963. However, it was only useful for prewashing up to 40 °C, since the bacterial enzymes used could not withstand greater temperatures.

This problem has been solved as well by selecting similar bacterial enzymes which were less sensitive to temperature and permitted rapid multiplication by way of fermentation. That was the beginning of enzyme detergents.

The first enzymatic detergent provided with almost as much heat stability as the enzymes in volcanic lava was marketed in 1967. It sometimes caused skin irritation and allergies, leading to several enzyme modifications and ultimately to its being banned. The biotechnological industry is still busy trying to find the optimal enzyme and to incorporate it into washing powder.

Naturally, protein-dissolving enzymes also play a large role in spot removal and dry cleaning. Also for cleaning sewage pipes, purification of drinking water, in the textile and leather industries, in the destruction of the masses of waste cellulose produced in the papermaking industry and in cleaning up oil spills, just to mention a few examples.

Enzyme production on demand

The successes of biotechnology to this point are remarkable. The subservient genie of the bottle is still not prepared to fulfill all of our wishes, but we are well on the way to taming ever more enzymes and reducing their sensitivity thanks to painstaking research (with the Japanese taking the lead here).

This task has succeeded mainly with the aid of microorganisms, a term which has already been mentioned several times. Microorganisms are microscopic animals and plants invisible to the naked eye. They include bacteria, viruses, molds, algae, and such single-celled species as amoebas, ciliates and many more. Sometimes it is even a mystery whether they are animals or plants. They all demonstrate simple enzymatic metabolism and are quite able to synthesize other enzymes. In addition, they sometimes release their enzymes freely into the environment which can then be filtered off easily.

Extremely sensitive enzymes can be bound to solids in the laboratory, thereby becoming immobilized. They are subsequently able to stand considerably rougher treatment and survive much longer. Biotechnologists have made the greatest advances in the field of immobilized enzymes, including mastery of the most important enzymatic processes.

The projects on which they are working sound fantastic. Do you still remember the frozen or dried-out baby shrimp? Professor Hand of the University of California in Davis has discovered what is behind this natural secret. He has investigated the embryos of this shrimp species which can withstand almost anything if they are frozen or dried out. They can be left lying about for years in the dry state, where they give an impression of being 'dead'. There are other life forms, some shellfish and desert plants, that fall into this state as well.

"When these organisms are allowed to remain desiccated over a longer period and are then put in water, they grow into perfect life forms. Just like instant coffee, when you add water you have aromatic coffee", explains Professor Hand. He discovered that these shrimp embryos store their enzymes in a viscous liquid containing *trehalose*, a sugar. This sugar syrup protects the enzymes from both cold and desiccation.

Professor Hand then dissolved other normally very temperature-sensitive enzymes in a trehalose/zinc solution, froze them, thawed them, refroze them and thawed them once again, and came to the conclusion that even repetition of this procedure caused almost no alteration in the enzymatic activity. It is likely that this new method will find many applications once its initial problems have been solved. It could make it possible to stabilize even the very temperature-sensitive insulin.

Reportedly, Genentec, a biotechnology corporation in San Francisco, is making use of genetic engineering to change the amino acids in the chains of digestive enzymes so that they lose their sensitivity to temperature and also to the surrounding acidic or basic environment. Other enzyme activities have also been changed. For example, instead of decomposing fats and oils, certain enzymes altered by genetic engineering are able to synthesize fats. They are able to convert inexpensive palm oil to cocoa butter or achieve other wonderful feats.

Once again: And there was light

Every advance is not necessarily a long awaited blessing for humanity. Sometimes, things everyone could do without are produced as by-products.There is a weakness in the bioluminescence story, for example. We do not know why the railroad worm of Uruguay glows in two colors, but we do know how it does this, i.e. the internal biotechnology of how it switches the light on.

In general, bioluminescence is always produced by the same mechanism; an enzyme taking its name from the devil, *luciferase*, catalyzes a reaction with oxygen to make a complex molecule known as *luciferin producellight*.

This procedure has been reproduced in the laboratory. Luciferin and luciferase have been extracted from fireflies and placed in a test tube with magnesium ions and an important biochemical energy source known as ATP (adenosine triphosphate). After mixing, the contents of the tube begin to glow.

Dr. David Ow of the University of California in San Diego is a specialist in this field. He is so skilled in handling luciferin and luciferase that he can easily make any organism he wishes glow. For instance, he incorporates the genetic information for luciferase into tobacco plants, places a tobacco seed in luciferin solution and the seed begins to germinate and glow with a mysterious green color.

This is not as pointless as it may sound. Since this method has been perfected, it has been possible to carry out tests as never before. Plants that have been thus treated to glow and subsequently multiply by cloning make it possible to see at a glance whether their genotype has been altered through mutation.

Marine biologists at the Scripps Institute of Oceanography in La Jolla, California have taken another path in the mastery of bioluminescence. They removed a self-luminescent gene package from the easier to handle microorganisms responsible for marine luminescence and then transferred this gene package known as LUX (which naturally contains luciferase and luciferin) into bacteria pathogenic to plants. The glow of infected plants makes it possible to follow exactly where the bacteria are. Biotechnological tricks such as this will naturally prove their worth in medical diagnostics as well.

Coincidentally, one of the by-products of these scientific achievements appears fascinating. American marine biologists believe it would be perfectly possible to introduce the LUX gene package into the flowers at the roadside or into Christmas trees so that we could then drive at night past mysteriously glowing flowers, or stand reverently beneath a Christmas tree that looked as if it had been colonized by a horde of glowworms.

Let us rather concern ourselves with a use of enzymes, since that is certain to be the main interest of the reader. The medicinal application of enzymes must concern the readers, for themselves and for their health.

Chapter 5

Medicine: A faithful servant

In the Bible, the 2nd Book of Kings, Chapter 20, it says, "At this time Hezekiah fell dangerously ill and the prophet Isiah son of Amoz came to him and said, `This is the word of the LORD: Give your last instructions to your household, for you are a dying man and will not recover'. Some theologians believe that King Hezekiah was suffering from cancer. He implored God in tears to spare him. The Lord heard him and, as the prophet was about to leave the citadel, said to Isiah that he had decided to make Hezekiah healthy again. Not only that, Hezekiah was to live for another fifteen years. "Then Isiah told them to apply a fig-plaster; so they made one and applied it to the boil, and he recovered."

If we accept that this was indeed cancer, then this is the oldest documented case of enzyme treatment for cancer leading to a presumed 'cure'. Afterall, medicine uses the term 'five-year cure', implying that it is the medical opinion that survival of cancer lasting a minimum of five years is a conditional 'cure'.

The primitive races of Africa, Asia, Australia and America also recognized this God-given remedy present in certain plants and used them for skin ulcers, wounds and other diseases (Figure 16). Some trickled the sap of the fig tree into the wounds and others laid the flesh of the papaya fruit or crushed fresh pineapples on them. These plants all contain large quantities of protein-dissolving enzymes, the proteases already mentioned. The Mayas, Aztecs and Incas used poultices prepared from plants (now known to be rich in enzymes) to treat various diseases. These included the 'medicine plant' (Aloe vera), papaya and pineapples.

Similar methods were also applied for hundreds of years in Europe by herb women, barber-surgeons and quacksalvers, simply because they helped. It was empirical medicine. At the time, nobody would have thought of refusing such treatment just because no one knew how it worked. Modern medicine often rejects certain treatments when a scientific explanation for how they work cannot be found. However, it is difficult to argue with results.

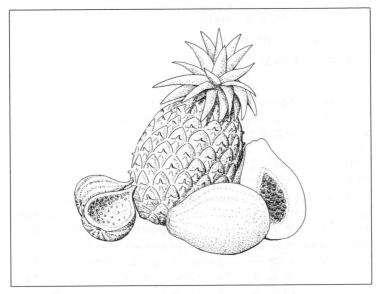

Figure 16: Papayas, figs and pineapples are especially rich in proteases

Nothing against research, it is important and provides us with ever more knowledge which we can apply to healing and the maintenance of health. We all would do well to support research in every possible way. For example, we have scientific research to thank for deciphering the first and long-unknown enzyme. The first of the busy and helpful sprites that do so much which is necessary for life.

Scientists naturally realized, even then, what fantastic opportunities there would be if these sprites could be trained to be obedient servants of medicine.

The previous century was therefore the era when we began to go beyond a blind, instinctive use to a targeted, deliberate exploitation of enzymes for medical purposes. The application of enzymes in medicine is divided roughly into three fields:

a) analysis and diagnosis

b) pharmacology

c) therapy

However, the story had a drawback from the start. In order to be able to use a particular enzyme in a targeted manner, it is first necessary to be able to isolate the enzymes individually. That did not prove to be easy. Many experiments failed and many theories remained just theories because the enzymes were not completely pure and absolutely free from other proteins.

Even today it is still one of the major tasks of enzymology to prepare purified enzymes in ever more perfect and economical ways. The better this succeeds, the greater the possible field of application and the more reliable the results.

Indeed, it is absolutely breath-taking what is now possible to achieve in the field of analysis with the aid of enzymes and it is a topic close to the hearts of biochemists, but practically every description of enzyme-controlled analysis would unfortunately be boring and cause nearly all readers to lay down this book with a sigh.

For the same reasons, the biotechnological applications of enzymes in pharmacology can only be dealt with here in a superficial manner. It should suffice to say that hundreds or even thousands of pharmacological substances can be prepared rapidly and reliably by the use of these obedient servants. This can be accomplished more quickly and more reliably than would be possible with normal chemical methods.

Many tons of insulin

The preparation of insulin for the diabetic forms a story all its own. The demand for this hormone is enormous. It has been estimated that there are over 120 million diabetics in the world, many of them requiring treatment with insulin. In the United States, over 14 million patients with diabetes are estimated (White). Of these, 10% or 1.4 million are insulin dependent type I diabetics and a little over 12 million are type II, 1/3 of whom also require insulin (4 million) for a combined total of nearly 6 million patients on insulin at a cost of more than $ 20 billion per year.

Diabetes is the seventh leading cause of death in the U.S. (about 150,000 deaths per year). Insulin is essential to life. The insulin required to treat millions of diabetics until recently was extracted from the pancreas of pigs and beef after slaughter. German sources estimate that in order to provide 100,000 patients with porcine insulin it is necessary to slaughter 3.5 million pigs. Likewise, in the United States over 20,000 tons of beef pancreas were required per year to supply the demand. In other words, it takes 14 cows' and 70 pigs' pancreas to supply a diabetic patient for one year. In 1984, 79 million animal pancreas were required to meet the U.S. needs. It was the last full year of animal derived pancreatic insulin. In recent years, the sources of animal pancreas have diminished considerably.

Traditionally, beef, pork and combinations of both have been preferred sources of insulin. In the United States, insulins from animal pancreas, particulary beef-pork combinations, are still used in 50% of all diabetics. In Europe, pig insulin was preferred, based on the concept that pigs are very similar to humans, at least at the physiological level, and the pork insulin has been shown to be less antigenic than beef. Unfortunately, porcine insulin is not quite the same as human insulin. Just one of the amino acids in the rather long amino acid chain is different from that of human insulin. This is where proteolytic enzymes come in. A specific cleavage process by means of an enzyme used pharmaceutically for just this purpose removes this amino acid which is typical of insulin from the pig, and a copy of human insulin is thus available.

However, purification presented real problems for a long period. When insulin production was first begun, it was still impossible to free the porcine insulin from all the foreign protein. The introduction of foreign protein into the human body can bring about potentially lethal allergic shock reactions. Only highly purified human insulin is used today.

Modern technology makes it possible to produce **biosynthetic** recombinant human type insulin derived from bacteria or from yeast, and **semisynthetic** human type insulin converted from pork.

Soon it will probably be possible to dispense with pigs and beef entirely. Japan and the United States deserve credit for much of the research and advances in this field. Genetic engineering has made it possible to train microorganisms to produce insulin. In recent years, an insulin identical to human insulin has been prepared from a microorganism known as E. coli, utilizing a method known as recombinant DNA technique. Here, the bacteria have been genetically altered by the addition of the human gene for insulin production. Two products are now commercially available for injections in the United States and marketed as 'Humulin' and 'Novolin'. They are widely used in the treatment of diabetic patients at present.

The desired error

The enzyme inhibitors which have already been discussed also play an extremely important role in pharmacology. We are not referring to the inhibitors made by our bodies to maintain the equilibrium of forces within them, but to a number of externally administered look-alike substances which are chemically very similar to the components used to produce essential coenzymes. These look-alike substances block the active site of the enzyme awaiting its coenzyme and inactivate it, sometimes forever.

Unfortunately, external, look-alike inhibitors can lead to specific damage in the organism because every artificial inhibition of an enzyme then interferes with some aspect of the body's metabolism. For this reason, such enzyme-inhibiting drugs as steroids (cortisone), cytostatics (anticancer agents for inhibiting cell division in cancer patients) or antibiotics (in English 'against life') always involve the risk of considerable side effects. In order to reduce these side effects as much as possible, they are usually prescribed to be taken for short periods of time, whenever possible. Administration over longer periods of time is generally considered only in exceptional situations when the danger or severity of the illness is so high that it justifies the risk of the medication.

It would, in fact, be more sensible in situations of illness to activate desired enzymes rather than to *inhibit undesired enzymes*. Pharmacology and medicine have achieved a great deal in this direction, but it has unfortunately found little application as yet. The principles will be explained in separate sections.

To know what one has – The art of diagnosis

Less explanation is necessary when describing enzyme-dependent diagnosis. The physician understands this subject inside out, although the patient understands little about what these strange units and levels are.

Only this much; at the start of this century, research workers, particularly the bacteriologist Wassermann and the internist Wohlgemuth, recognized how much information could be obtained concerning bodily disorders by measuring the activities of specific enzymes. Wassermann was able to establish the presence of syphilis with the aid of animal enzymes; with Wohlgemuth's research, it has been possible to use the activity of the body's own enzymes to diagnose pancreatitis (inflammation of the pancreas) with a high degree of certainty.

This ingenious method of obtaining rapid and reliable diagnostic information by measuring the activities of enzymes in the blood, the cerebrospinal fluid, the amniotic fluid, saliva, pancreatic secretions, gastric juices, urine and body tissues has become an indispensable part of the physician's daily work. It has brought about a revolution in diagnosis.

Previously, for instance, time-consuming chemical reactions were required to measure the concentration of sugar in a patient's blood. It was complicated, took at least two hours and the blood sugar level obtained was imprecise. Today, the determination is completed in a few minutes and the result is accurate. Anyone prepared to lay out a few cents for a test strip to determine the sugar in his or her urine will confirm this.

Enzymatic diagnosis can be refined even further, since it is now known that individual enzymes concentrate themselves in the various organs according to a particular pattern. So-called *enzyme profiles* are presently available from which one can see whether something is abnormal or not.

Almost all of the 3,000 or more enzymes which might be in our organism are to be found in our bloodstream. For this reason, the activity of the enzymes in a sample of blood will remain the most common diagnostic tool for a long time to come.

Correcting errors

In addition to enzymatic analysis, diagnosis and pharmacology, it has naturally been considered how these biotechnologically-conjured servants might also provide their services for therapy.

A new era in enzyme therapy was thus begun. It has been applied to correct metabolic disorders, i.e. to correct disturbances of organ function or cell formation, to correct metabolically-developed intoxications and to repair genetic defects.

Scientists soon concluded, from the knowledge they collected concerning enzymes as tools for the assembly of living material, that genetic defects required the application of enzymes to either correct or neutralize them. In addition, genetic defects are almost always enzyme defects as well.

More than 200 different diseases resulting from genetically-dependent enzyme defects have already been described in the medical literature. Either the patient's body does not produce some particular enzyme at all or it produces a similar although much less active enzyme instead.

Incidentally, every human being and indeed, every nonhuman primate, is born with one enzymatic defect since humans and other primates, in contrast to all other mammals, cannot produce the enzyme *uricase*. This uricase serves the important function of decomposing uric acid. We are unable to achieve the removal of uric acid as well as the other mammals and attempt to carry out the process laboriously with a substitute enzyme. The result is that humans and nonhuman primates occasionally produce excessive amounts of insufficiently decomposed uric acid salts, and deposit them in their bodies, usually in and around their joints – an illness known as gout.

A number of disorders of red cell metabolism are due to hereditary enzyme deficiencies, and defects that interfere with the energy source of the red cells which might also lead to anemia. Other defects contribute to abnormal red cell membranes and also result in abnormal red blood cells and subsequent anemia. The normal adult hemoglobin (HbA) consists of two principal pairs of polypeptide chains known as alpha and beta. Abnormalities in these chains can result in anemia as well. Enzymes are very important in the proper function and metabolism of hemoglobin.

Some genetically determined enzyme defects are found primarily in the humans of one race. For example, the black population is affected more frequently by a genetically determined defect which can lead to *sickle cell anemia*. The defect is due to the inheritance of an abnormal form of hemoglobin. This 'hemoglobin S' differs from the normal hemoglobin A in that valine is substituted for glutamic acid in the sixth amino acid position of its beta chain. The defect causes the hemoglobin to distort when the oxygen concentration is low. At low oxygen concentrations, the abnormal hemoglobin causes an alteration in the red cells which results in a sickle shape. These abnormally shaped cells are inflexible, plug smaller blood vessels and lead to serious occlusion. In addition, they are too fragile and break down easily (hemolysis), resulting subsequently in anemia. Enzyme defects are felt to contribute to the production of this abnormal 'hemoglobin S'.

It has also been reported that half of certain oriental ethnic groups suffer from a 'genetically-transmitted metabolic defect', as such defects have also been called, which leads to an extreme *sensitivity to alcohol*. They produce too little *aldehyde dehydrogenase*, the enzyme extensively responsible for the degradation of alcohol. After alcohol consumption, the concentration of one of the metabolic products of alcohol increases because of the lacking alcohol degradation due to this enzyme defect. This substance leads to hyper-intensive reactions, unexpected outbursts, increased excitability and malaise. This is the explanation as to why some oriental persons who seldom reveal signs of emotion in the absence of alcohol appear to be completely out of control after drinking alcohol and behave in a very uncharacteristic manner. It also explains why so many orientals are total abstainers, due to the knowledge of this reaction which causes them to lose control. Furthermore, it explains why some women have less tolerance for alcohol than men, since women also have very little of this enzyme.

Genetically-transmitted enzyme defects differ greatly in the severity of their consequences. The effects of some are barely noticed, some are accountable for a considerable amount of disease and a few are lethal, particularly in babies and children.

At present, conservative medicine concentrates on preventing or stopping some of the consequences of these defects by manipulating the diet and similar methods. Recent advances in medicine aim at repair of the enzyme defect by enzymatic measures, although thus far with limited success.

Genetic enzymatic defects – Poisons and antidotes

The consequences of these genetic disorders are usually the result of the accumulation and deposition of substances which are not assimilated due to the enzymatic defect. These act as poisons in the body. Some advances in detoxification have been made with the aid of enzymes.

The treatment of poison gas victims is a well-known example. One of the most terrible poison gases is dichlorodiethyl sulfide, also known as *mustard gas*. It functions by enzymatically inhibiting the transmission of nerve impulses. Surprisingly, a species of squid possesses just the enzyme that is capable of destroying the enzyme-inhibitor in mustard gas. The enzyme in squids has been isolated and can, if used in time, save the lives of mustard gas victims.

Another example involves the dialysis necessary in the event of kidney damage. In order to spare kidney patients the lengthy and expensive process of dialysis, intensive efforts are being made to manufacture small artificial kidneys. They are already functional for animals. Scaled up for human use, an artificial kidney prototype consists of a tube about ten centimeters in length and two centimeters in diameter connected to a kidney through the abdominal wall. The tube is filled with the enzyme urease bound to carbon. These bonded enzymes are surrounded by nylon microcapsules to delay their release and allow them to be transported slowly into the kidney. That would be a primitive model of a kidney, but it could well suffice to spare kidney patients the usual dialysis for removing some of the toxic metabolic residues from the body.

Thus, an artificial kidney is within the realms of the possible. However, we will have to wait quite some time for the arrival of the artificial liver since the liver is a very complex biochemical factory absolutely packed with enzymes. The construction of this factory is still beyond man's capabilities.

Nevertheless, it is possible to imitate one of the liver's functions, since the enzymes in the liver which function in removing some metabolic poisons are known. Utilizing genetic engineering, fragments containing the active templates or 'plans' of some known detoxifying enzymes have been genetically implanted into microorganisms which then produce them industriously. They can then be used to remove metabolic wastes from the liver by breaking the poisons down and making them more water-soluble. These poisons can then be excreted from the body by natural routes. At present, however, there are still difficulties in activating such biochemically-produced liver enzymes after their introduction into our metabolism.

Considering the relatively short time period which has elapsed since the initial experiments in the field of enzyme therapy, the scientists concerned can pat themselves on the back and be hopeful that they will have made great strides by the end of the century.

Clearing the pipes

Conventional medicine has had its greatest success to date in the enzymatic treatment of circulatory disturbances. More accurately, in dissolving blood clots which are known as thrombi.

For this reason, thrombolysis, the dissolution of thrombi, is also a favorite topic of enzymologists. Without going into the important but somewhat complicated story of blood-flow equilibrium, it is sufficient to say here that blood platelets can adhere to one another for various reasons and cause the growth of blood clots on the walls of the arteries and veins which threaten to close these vessels. This can lead to many painful and dangerous developments. Thus, a lethal embolism can occur if they are transported into a narrow vessel. Heart attacks too are usually provoked by thrombi in the arteries of the heart.

It is no wonder that every effort is made to cause the thrombi to dissolve, to promote thrombolysis (Figures 17 and 37). In our bodies, an enzyme called *plasmin* is responsible for this thrombolysis. It is present in large quantities in our blood, mainly in an inactive state because the 'safety catch' is still on. The enzyme is known as *plasminogen* in this inactive form and has to be armed like a weapon. This activation of the plasminogen determines to what extent and how rapidly thrombi are dissolved. Therefore, the dissolution of dangerous thrombi is always dependent on the activation of plasminogen.

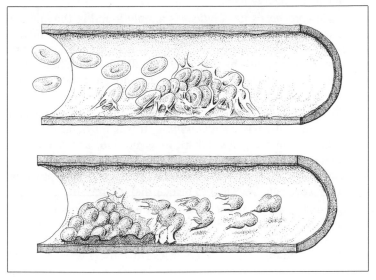

Figure 17:   Above: Red blood cells adhere to one another and form a clot on the vessel walls
Below: Thrombolysis: Dissolution of a blood clot

Plasminogen can be activated fully to plasmin by means of a plasminogen activator. Plasminogen activators are, and this will no longer surprise you, special enzymes. These enzymes can either be introduced into the circulating blood by infusion, or introduced directly to the site of the blood clot by means of a catheter. Their only task is to react with inactive plasminogen, removing its safety catch, and changing it into active plasmin. Plasmin then dissolves the thrombus specifically and everything is in order.

The enzymatic dissolution of blood clots is also known as fibrinolysis. The first fibrinolytic used in conventional medical practice for thrombolysis was obtained from the coccobacterium *Streptococcus hemolyticus*.

This *Streptococcus hemolyticus* is mainly found in the mucosa of the mouth and can cause tonsillitis, scarlet fever or an inflammation of the middle ear. Of all things, this particular bacterium possesses a coenzyme which is capable of fibrinolysis. That is, it is capable of converting the inactive plasminogen present in the blood into active plasmin.

This coenzyme has been removed from the streptococci and therefore given the name *streptokinase*. It was introduced for the first time in America, more than 40 years ago, as an infusion intended to activate plasminogen. In this way, a final victory over all coagulation diseases was hoped for, ranging from closure of the leg arteries (smoker's leg) to myocardial infarction.

The jubilation was somewhat premature. Many people were found to have already built up antibodies to streptococci as a result of prior infections. This can lead to side effects when streptokinase is administered intravenously. Thus, there were frequent allergic shock reactions when streptokinase was administered because it was not yet known how to free streptokinase from all traces of foreign proteins and thereby apply it in its purest form.

The breakthrough was first made by the German company, Hoechst, in 1962 when a stabilized high purity streptokinase was marketed for pharmaceutical application. It was infused by intravenous drip over a period of hours into the bloodstream of thrombotic patients or directly applied to the site of the thrombus using a catheter.

The medical world was still not entirely satisfied. The ability of this streptokinase to activate plasminogen was still too weak and there were also some problems with the exact control of the equilibrium between thinning of the blood and blood coagulation. A particular complication could occur if too much plasminogen was activated, resulting in plasminogen depletion.

The kidneys as a source

An enzyme we steadfastly excrete in the urine, which therefore received the name *urokinase*, was discovered in the search for an even better and more powerful plasminogen activator. Urokinase is an excellent fibrinolytic, it interacts with plasminogen and activates it directly to plasmin. The activated plasmin then selectively attacks the sticky protein of the thrombus and dissolves the blood clot. The danger of the blood vessel being stuck together or blocked by thrombi is thereby averted.

Nevertheless, urokinase, like streptokinase, must also be administered in the hospital by infusion or directly into the vessel by means of a catheter. However, there are fewer risks of allergy or intolerance.

The problem this time is rather in the production of urokinase, since the fact that we incessantly excrete urokinase in the urine does not mean this happens in quantities worth mentioning. All of 29 milligrams of purified urokinase can be isolated from 2,300 liters of urine. This naturally made its initial use rather expensive. Only recently has it been possible to cultivate cell tissue obtained from kidneys in the laboratory and, using biotechnological tricks, to persuade it to produce urokinase.

However, physicians were still not satisfied. The administration of urokinase in patients with thromboses remained a complicated and expensive procedure that could only be performed in the hospital. Therefore, the search continued for other enzymes which might be better at activating plasminogen, safer and easier to administer. Tests were made on animals that produce venoms which function via the enzymatic dissolution of proteins in blood. Experiments were made with bee, toad and snake venoms. In certain cases, they may indeed be applied pharmacologically, although they are less suitable for the control of plasminogen activation.

Attempts were made to dissolve thrombi with *hyaluronidase* as well. This is a special protein-dissolving enzyme obtainable from various sources. Among other things, one must thank hyaluronidase for our development since the sperm of every man is provided with hyaluronidase from the testicles. The function of hyaluronidase is to dissolve the proteinaceous coating of the female ovum, thereby making the penetration of the sperm and fertilization of the egg cell possible.

A recent form of enzymatic thrombolysis in the ever developing therapy involves the use of *TPA (tissue plasminogen activator)*, a rapid, relatively safe plasminogen activator. Every hospital emergency room in the United States, Germany and most countries has TPA and the equipment for its infusion, so that in the event of cardiac infarction, the medical team can then infuse it and very probably save the life of the patient. They also have other thrombolytic agents. Eventually, most ambulances will be similarly equipped.

Enzymes by mouth?

The obvious question is whether we can consume enzymes to improve our health and the answer is, "Yes!". We do it virtually every day. We consume a great deal of enzymes with our food and these contribute to keeping us healthy. Enzymes are everywhere, in herbs, onions, garlic, curds and yoghurt. In addition to helping us with a healthy digestion, other benefits have been discovered by scientists.

Since most readers who already know something about enzymes probably associate these with digestion, this topic deserves a short chapter of its own.

Chapter 6

Digestion: A means to live

No matter what we eat, grilled T-bone steak and Idaho potatoes, chocolate cake with whipped cream or crispbread with radishes, we consume nothing more and nothing less than proteins, carbohydrates and fats.

In order to convert these three basic food materials into biochemical substances that we can use, we need three groups of enzymes, the protein-decomposing 'proteolytic' enzymes (*proteases*), the fat-decomposing 'lipolytic' enzymes (*lipases*), and the carbohydrate-decomposing 'amylolytic' enzymes (*amylases*) (Figure 18).

This enzymatic transformation starts as soon as we take the first bite, since even when it is being chewed the food is being controlled by the amylases in the saliva to see if there is work to be done for them, i.e. whether there are carbohydrates to be broken down and processed. Our bodies have a certain preference for carbohydrates, the digestive system acts on them first, then on the proteins and finally on the fats.

Let us follow the food from the mouth on its way to further processing. The food, hopefully well-chewed, is mixed to a paste with the saliva and transported through the esophagus into the stomach. The better the food has been broken down and mixed with the saliva, the better for the stomach. First of all, it accepts the consignment from the esophagus and then sends signals by means of certain hormones to the gallbladder and the pancreas, requesting them to make sufficient enzymes available for the work to be performed in the intestinal tract.

In addition, the amylases to be found in the stomach proceed with the activity on the carbohydrates initiated by their colleagues in the saliva. At the same time, the proteins present in the food paste are decomposed. For this purpose, the stomach produces

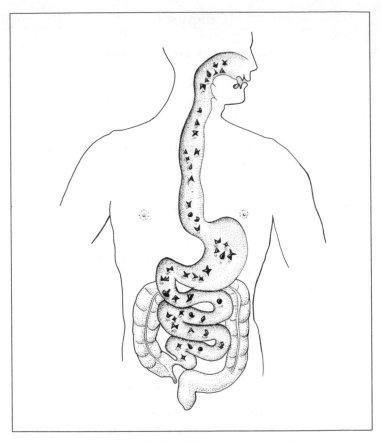

Figure 18: A great number of enzymes in the gastrointestinal tract are responsible
            for digestion

between one and two liters of gastric juice each day containing
primarily hydrochloric acid and several protein-degrading
enzymes such as *pepsin* and *cathepsin*. Babies also produce the

enzyme *chymosin (rennin)*, which is of special importance for the utilization of milk protein.

Cathepsins deserve special mention. They are naturally present in the animal tissues we eat. The richest sources are liver, kidney and spleen, but they are also present in the various forms of meat and fish we consume. They are located primarily within the lysosomal fraction of the cells of these tissues. They are naturally released when these foods age and are responsible to a large extent for their decomposition. When the tissues are eaten fresh, the cathepsins are initially released after the action of the hydrochloric acid in the stomach, but their release continues as the digestion progresses in the duodenum and rest of the bowel.

Our own internal cathepsins are important in the breakdown of damaged tissues, as after injuries or wounds, and possibly in the breakdown of undesired cells, such as early cancerous cells. Although a number of cathepsins are known, five principal types have been isolated. These are cathepsins B, C, D, G and L. Cathepsin B hydrolyses protein with a specificity resembling papain. In addition to digestion, cathepsin C enhances the proteolysis of prothrombin to thrombin. Cathepsin D is important in the metabolism of cartilage and connective tissue. It also resembles pepsin A in its actions. Cathepsin G has catalytical as well as chymotrypsin-like properties. According to Starkey et al, it is also most important in relation to its immunological properties. Cathepsin L is important in the hydrolysis of proteins.

The protein-degrading enzymes are first activated by the hydrochloric acid so that these proteases are able to function. The hydrochloric acid is also important in that it stimulates hormone production in the stomach, destroys some of the bacteria present in the food paste and promotes the uptake of minerals and trace elements into the bloodstream, some of which serve as coenzymes.

The pylorus of the stomach releases the stomach contents in portions into the proximal portion of the small intestine, the duodenum (in simple English 'twelve-finger gut'), so-called because it is about twelve finger-breadths in length, as physicians already discovered a few hundred years ago. Nowadays, medicine has become a more exact science and cannot afford to associate itself with such rough estimates.

Many people believe that the stomach is the main site of food processing, but, although very important, this is simply not true. The most thorough activities are performed in the duodenum. For this reason, it is important that the stomach has already sent signals to the hormone system that work can be expected. This ensures that the intestines receive enough secretion from the pancreas. Aside from such hormones as *insulin* and *glucagon*, the pancreas also provides about a liter and a half of digestive juices for the duodenum each day.

This contains essentially the three groups of enzymes already mentioned:

*   *Proteolytic enzymes (proteases)*:
    These include *trypsin, chymotrypsin* as well as the *peptidases*, *elastases* and *cathepsins*. They are capable of degrading up to 300 g protein per hour.

*   *Lipolytic enzymes (lipases)*:
    These can degrade up to 175 g fat per hour. In order to make this possible, the fat is first brought into solution by the bile, i.e. the liquid from the gallbladder. This solubilization of the fat is known as emulsification.

*   *Amylolytic enzymes (amylases)*:
    These are able to degrade up to 300 g carbohydrate per hour.

Prepared for absorption

When the food substances have been so altered by the enzymes in the duodenum that they now consist of minute fragments which can readily be used by the body, they are transported to the next two sections of the small intestine, the jejunum and ileum. It is principally here that usable components are taken up by the body. They are absorbed.

Absorption in these sections of the small intestine proceeds rather like sorting out specific parts from a conveyor belt. Individual substances are selected along the entire length of the small intestine and transported through the wall into the circulatory system.

Naturally, if the absorption through the wall of the small intestine into the bloodstream is disturbed, the whole digestive system soon ceases to function. This has repercussions on the stomach and the affected person suffers from gastrointestinal discomforts.

No one will now be surprised to learn that enzymes play a decisive role in the absorption of building components from the intestinal tract into the circulatory system. Furthermore, numerous enzymes are essential as transporters for useful substances that the body needs.

The nonusable components remain in the intestines as waste products. The water is withdrawn, and they are thickened, pass into the large intestine and finally end in the rectum as stool. A certain amount of subtle utilization can even occur here, since the entire digestive tract, particularly the large intestine and rectum, is alive with independent microorganisms that are able to seek out sufficient nutrition for their own purposes from the already substantially exploited food residues.

They are foreign organisms that have settled in our bowels as friendly, well-behaved parasites. Strange to say, our bodies do not try to combat these parasitic organisms, although as foreign bodies they ought to be recognized and combated by our immune systems. Interestingly enough, a truce has been called here, the understanding of which could be of use in solving the problem of rejection after organ transplantation.

Our body makes this exception in the case of the foreign bacteria, the intestinal flora, because it profits from their presence. It is a mutual benefit society, a symbiosis. During the digestive processes of these bacteria, by-products are formed that our bodies can well utilize. An example is the vitamin K mandatory for blood coagulation. It has also been suggested that microorganisms present in the bowel, may also be important in the final enzyme-assisted absorption of certain vitamins and medications. For example, the destruction of the microorganisms by antibiotics can contribute to vitamin B6 deficiency, or can lead to interference with the absorption of birth control pills.

Incidentally, some of these organisms are capable of biolumi-nescence, the enzymatically produced 'cold' light we have already discussed. Weak lamps are thus continually illuminating our bowels.

Eat more enzymes!

In addition to the three basic food materials protein, fat and carbohydrate, we also consume small quantities of other substances: Vitamins, minerals and trace elements. Of interest, the alcohol we consume also plays a special role.

The naturally occurring enzymes we eat in fresh and raw foods are also of great importance. What enzymes these are and in what quantity depends on the type of food and the state in which the food is eaten. For instance, fresh, naturally-ripened pineapples are rich in the protein-splitting enzyme *bromelain*, although scarcely any can be found in canned pineapples.

In learning to heat and cook foods, our forefathers have probably done our tongues and teeth a favor, but they have done less for our digestive systems and health since heating destroys virtually all the enzymes in our food.

Neither has the food industry always done everything in its power to preserve the health value of foods. The products with no life in them at all include so-called super-fine flour and refined sugar. They are 'empty' carbohydrates or food skeletons, which contribute to many of the diseases of modern civilization from which we presently suffer.

We cannot expect fast-food restaurants to stop selling french fries, ketchup, white buns and cola in consideration of our enzyme requirements. Neither is it to be expected that we will stop grilling meat or otherwise turn from less healthy to more healthy foods.

Nevertheless, something would be gained if we were to eat something fresh or raw with each meal. For example, much can be gained if we begin our main meals with a plate of salad with carrots, fennel, leeks, beets or celery; if we were to lightly steam our vegetables, and if we were to use salt sparingly – a substance which acts an indirect enzyme inhibitor; or if we were to serve meat which is difficult to digest with such enzyme-rich foods as raw sauerkraut, onions, garlic or fresh herbs to aid digestion.

Some oriental cultures also have an instinctive sense for healthy nutrition. They eat enzyme-rich foods, such as raw fish and raw seafood, hopefully from unpolluted waters, and they eat meat with relatively large quantities of soy sauce.

Soy sauce is perhaps the oldest 'enzyme agent' of all. Its digestion-promoting properties have been recognized in Asia for thousands of years. It is prepared by mixing soy flour with barley or rice which is then fermented with the aid of a fungus. This fungus (*Aspergillus oryzae*) contains highly active enzymes which have been given the name *pronases*. The pronases in soy sauce, which is only ready for use after years of fermentation (the famous Worcestershire sauce is no different in principle), retain their power which then is applied for the breakdown of meat protein. A hybrid of this fungus has now been developed in Japan so that what may be called *super-pronases* can be attained.

Unfortunately, we do not generally eat what our instinct and common sense tell us to. We do not eat the right quantities of the right foods at the right times and in the proper manner. The results can include digestive disturbances, deposition of fat, and becoming overweight. These findings can be associated with further health problems including disorders of the circulation which lead to more severe cardiovascular disease and disorders of the heart. The reducing diets often recommended generally provide only temporary weight loss and many of them may even be more detrimental to health in the long run. Likewise, administration of laxatives for weight loss usually produce only short-term improvements, if any, and in fact may be harmful in the long run.

Aid for the digestion

We should all eat properly and follow a balanced diet containing a substantial amount of fresh foods in each meal. We should also avoid highly processed, skeletonized foods and high levels of preservatives, additives or chemicals such as insecticides, fungicides, etc. If we are unable to do this, we can take natural digestive enzymes in order to support our overtaxed digestive apparatus. There are dozens of preparations of this type. *Pepsin wine* is probably the best-known, it contains the enzyme pepsin which is essential for protein digestion.

We probably ought to pay more attention to brewer's yeast as well, since the cells of fresh brewer's yeast make copious quantities of vitamins, minerals and trace elements available to our bodies which stimulate enzyme activity in the intestines, equivalent to a 'spring cleaning'. Harmful bacteria are removed and replaced by health-giving bacteria. This spring cleaning of the bowels can be intensified by eating such preparations as yogurt which contain the useful microorganisms, the helpful foreign guests, of the intestinal flora.

Most of the enzyme preparations prescribed or obtained from the pharmacy and drug store for digestive disturbances, a bloated feeling, belching, flatulence, constipation or diarrhea are obtained from the pancreatic juice of pigs and contain many enzymes capable of breaking down proteins, fats and carbohydrates. Some of these preparations are also enriched enzyme agents such as ox bile, the products of the fungus *Aspergillus oryzae* or other aids.

Many preparations of this type are protected by a coating from the action of hydrochloric acid in the stomach, so that their activity can fully unfold in the small intestine. They aid the enzymes provided by the pancreas which are often overtaxed, particularly in the elderly, since the sins and abuses of bad diet are cumulative and lead to a gradual decrease in the body's own enzyme production. Abuses also contribute to an enlarged pancreas and liver.

These over-the-counter and prescription preparations often provide good digestive services, particularly in the small intestine. Shouldn't they also be effective throughout the whole body? For many of them this is impossible because they are not able to be absorbed and penetrate into the entire body. They are unable to journey along the exquisite pathway through the wall of the small intestine into the bloodstream and the lymph tract. They cannot function although enzymes are surely required more urgently and in greater quantities throughout the body for its metabolic processes than in the digestive tract.

Is it therefore impossible to simply swallow enzymes and make them available for the whole body? As mentioned earlier, this misconception is found to be widespread, even among physicians.

Help for the entire organism

Something scientists have dreamed of for a long time is that instead of having to painstakingly provide the body with the enzymes it requires by means of an infusion, with all the complications and limitations involved, is to be able to make enzymes available to the whole body by mouth, just like other drugs. What possibilities are there? A person suffering from a deficiency of a particular enzyme could simply swallow this missing helper. If a patient has a greatly increased requirement for a perfectly functioning enzyme, it would also be simple to prescribe this enzyme. Every disorder basically involves disturbed enzyme function with increased enzyme requirements, and it would be ideal to be able to replace it.

Many scientists have dreamed of this possibility, taken one look in their textbooks, sighed and rejected it. Afterall, the textbooks state quite clearly, "Enzymes are not absorbed by mouth. Unfortunately, it does not work. It cannot function."

We can swallow enzymes, indeed we ingest them every day with our food. According to the textbooks, "a limited deliberate enzyme therapy can be performed *within* the digestive tract by taking enzymes. But that is all, since enzymes are such high molecular mass proteins, they cannot pass through the narrow intestinal villi to reach the bloodstream and the lymph tract, and hence cannot reach the rest of the body." According to the older textbooks, "absorption of intact enzymes into the rest of the body is not possible." The sooner we correct these textbooks the better!

Rather, what is most exciting to scientists worldwide is the research during the past three decades, particularly the last decade, indicating that oral administration of specific enzymes can have systemic absorption and systemic effects on the whole organism. Of great interest are the numerous published reports in ethical medical journals worldwide, of clinical and scientific studies detailing the results of numerous trials utilizing systemically administered enzymes for various medical conditions. The studies were initially conducted in Europe and subsequently worldwide. The published results and experiences appear to substantially support their stated claim that it is possible to effectively and rationally treat certain chronic medical disorders with systemically administered enzymes. Today!

That is probably the most important statement in this whole book. The next chapter, where this statement is examined in some detail, should therefore be read carefully. We are talking about a unique concept previously not properly recognized in the United States, but widely used in Europe, Japan, China and other countries. The proposed concept advocates systemic enzyme therapy which is already being administered today. In addition to numerous clinical trials in progress, these treatments are at present legally prescribed in many countries and administered by physicians to millions of patients a year.

The collective published experiences of these trials and treatments suggest their value in the treatment of a number of conditions. These include certain chronic degenerative disorders, cancer, viral diseases and old age maladies. Most remarkable in these clinical studies were the repeated reports that the treatments with orally administered enzymes were virtually free of serious side effects.

Because the results are so encouraging and so many patients are under treatment worldwide, the authors felt that it was worthwhile to bring this information to the attention of the American public, in order to generate further interest and research on the subject. A treatment which is used so widely in so many countries, which is prescribed as an ethical and effective treatment by thousands of physicians worldwide, and which appears remarkably safe, can no longer be ignored in this country. We are talking about the health and maintenance of life of each and every person.

Chapter 7

Enzyme therapy: The European experience

A person is ill. No matter what is wrong, the first thing to understand is that something is out of order with his or her enzymes. Had the pertinent body enzymes succeeded in removing the causes of the health disturbance and maintained the body in its normal state of enzymatic balance, the person would not have become ill in the first place. For a long time, scientists have considered it logical that more enzymes of the required type and in the right quantity ought to be made available for almost every illness in order to end the disturbance in health. The new enzymes are needed in order to come to the aid of their weak, inferior, or perhaps even ailing enzyme colleague-in-arms.

European scientists have suggested that enzymes are important in disease prevention. Some feel that, "it is logical and sensible to take enzymes prophylactically as well, in order to have the fighting troops ready when a danger to health and therefore an increased enzyme requirement would be likely, for threatening colds to everyday sport's injuries."

This group of scientists also point out that, "ideally you take a handful of enzyme tablets, swallow them and the fresh auxiliary troops are already active. The guardians of health are now able to do their work." Furthermore, they state, "if rapid help is needed or large quantities are required, enzyme preparations can ideally be injected intramuscularly, subcutaneously, intravenously or administered as a microenema."

Is this really possible? Or is it just pie in the sky? Where is the flaw in our reasoning that makes this beautiful dream collapse like a house of cards?

First of all, many scientists feel that it is actually quite possible. Scientists are certainly not too far from being able to supply many of the 3,000 or more enzymes of the body in tablet form. European scientists propose that one can at present take a mixture of certain specific and important enzymes that demonstrate anti-inflammatory effects. They feel that the long-term damages from persistent unrelieved inflammation can be prevented in this way. They claim that these enzymes strengthen the body's own defenses, which help combat viruses and other infections, and have a number of other unique actions on the body. According to them, these enzymes have an important effect on inflammatory processes, they provide for a good blood supply, they help heal wounds and they even have a regulatory effect on the growth of degenerate cells. That is an impressive program, particularly if they can also help poorly responsive medical problems, such as those designated as chronic degenerative disorders.

Why not immediately?

The administration of such enzyme mixtures for the treatment of diseases of this type and as a precaution against them has been practiced, reportedly with considerable success, for more than 40 years. The question which naturally arises is why such a basic, versatile, seemingly successful method has not long since become standard medical practice. Why don't we all keep these remarkable health-givers in the bathroom next to the toothbrush glass ready for use?

The reason for this is the prevailing medical dogma or reasoning. Conventional medical practitioners have assimilated this persistent dogma and generally do not understand or accept systemic oral enzyme therapy. That has led to a negative and a closed widespread attitude. "It cannot be true or we all would be doing it", they reason.

So let us try to look at this dogma objectively and to understand the nature of this prejudice, because systemic enzyme therapy, if indeed as successful and functional as claimed in other countries, should be studied and properly judged in this country.

This brings us to the first objection, what is meant here by 'systemic' enzyme therapy? Put precisely, the infusion of urokinase or other enzymes into the circulatory system via the antecubital vein is a systemic therapy. Here, the enzymes reach all parts of the system. Certainly the representatives of 'systemic enzyme therapy' and of conventional academic medicine can probably agree that intravenous thrombolytic enzymes are indeed 'systemic enzymes'. For the Europeans, however, systemic can also apply to orally administered enzymes.

The difference to other uses of enzymes lies principally in what is known as the 'peroral' phase of enzyme therapy. That is the administration of enzymes by mouth with the resulting absorption into the circulatory system and hence into the whole body system.

If we omit the purely instinctive or traditional usage of enzymes from plant and other origins, utilized by primitive people and the ancient civilizations, the peroral phase began about 45 years ago.

First of all, some scientists in the United States decided to ignore accepted conventional theory and began to treat various inflammatory processes and blood coagulation disorders with oral enzymes by administering such suitable drugs as, for instance, trypsin or streptokinase. They felt that the effect was not so distinct as after intravenous infusion, but it was safer and easier to perform.

In Germany, it was the biochemist Gaschler who reported the successful treatment of certain forms of cancer by orally administering individual enzymes as drugs in 1937. The concept of using enzymes to treat cancer was not new. The Mayas and other people had already done so unwittingly when, for example, they treated malignant ulcers by applying papaya leaves and papaya juice. The enzyme *papain* contained in the papaya plant is a powerfully acting agent which breaks down 'unhealthy' protein. As early as the beginning of the present century, the physician Dr. Beard had injected pancreatic juice from freshly slaughtered calves into his cancer patients, producing such sensational success that he was taken for a charlatan. At the time, other scientists repeated the studies but used older pancreatic juice which no longer contained any active enzymes, because they had denatured due to aging of the solution, improper storage and contamination.. Of course it no longer worked, but unfortunately this lock of effect when denatured sufficed to scientifically refute the effectiveness of enzyme therapy for cancer. This will be described in more detail in the chapter on cancer and also in the following section on the role played by an extraordinary man. Let us pause for a moment with the certainly interesting, but nevertheless for some readers rather dry, biochemical discussion of enzymes.

A quite extraordinary man

He was possibly one of the last universal scientists in his thinking and in his work. Like a character in a novel. Let us briefly go into the story of his life. It will also make it easier to understand how the development of what is known as 'systemic' enzyme therapy evolved.

The person concerned is Max Wolf, (Figure 19) rather unobtrusive in appearance, only five foot one, with a powerful skull topped by a thin fringe of hair. Not necessarily a handsome man from the Hollywood standpoint, but he possessed a strong personality which made others around him seem colorless as soon as he entered the room. There are people who only met him briefly and who swear today that he was a giant and not a rather small man. He acted like a magnet to the most beautiful women, the cleverest scientists, the most famous artists and the mightiest politicians. They hung on to his every word and followed his every action.

His life is closely interwoven with the natural history and politics of our century. Born in 1885 as the son of a nationalistic German father and a Jewish mother in the strife-ridden Vienna of the still resplendent Austro-Hungarian Empire, he grew up in Bohemia (the Czech Republic) and left the no longer harmonious parental home, of his own accord, at the age of twelve. He took a train from Bohemia to Vienna and, once there, earned his living as a tutor of rich but unpromising fellow schoolboys. He made it through school quicker than the rest, studying structural and civil engineering. As an engineer, he made a number of technical discoveries of various kinds. He was, for instance, awarded patents for a technical installation which automatically stopped wrongly-switched railway trains. He then became bored with technology and developed his astonishing talent for drawing and painting. He became an artist and in a very short time was awarded the title of Court Painter to Emperor Franz Joseph of Austria.

At the outbreak of the First World War, the 29-year-old imperial court painter Max Wolf happened to be in New York visiting his brother. He remained, more or less unwillingly, in New York, since he would rather have joined the imperial army to serve at the front. Because of the war, he was stranded in New York City, and since his brother had studied medicine, he too began medical studies and after only a few semesters was giving lectures of his own at the university. This remarkable man already knew more than many of the professors who taught him.

Shortly after he completed his studies, he was invited to lecture on medical topics and was appointed professor of medicine at Fordham University in New York. He was awarded seven different doctorates during his lifetime. In addition to his duties as a university professor, he opened a medical practice together with his brother, trained himself as a gynecologist and ran the largest maternity center in the middle of the Italian and black districts of New York, in which more than 4,000 births were registered each year. On weekends, Wolf worked in addition, as an ear, nose and throat specialist. He was particularly interested in the hormone-secreting glands. Since not a single textbook on the hormone system was to be found in all of the medical literature, he sat down and wrote a textbook on endocrinology. It became a best seller, and his brother, to whom he had ceded the copyright, promptly

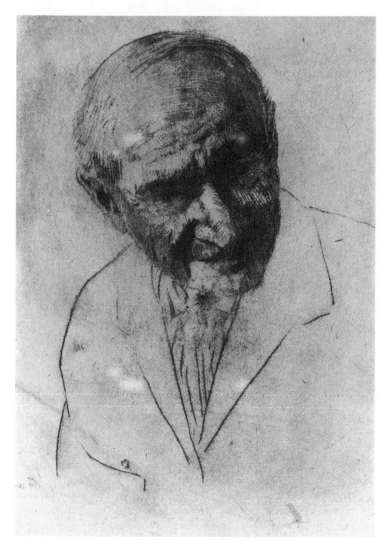

Figure 19: Professor Max Wolf, MD – the 'father' of therapeutic enzymes

became a millionaire, and that really meant something in those days.

Protein and a blue rose

Max Wolf, as his friends knew him, had other things on his mind than to mourn this million. He had struck out into a new scientific field, that of applied genetics. He undertook research in this field under his own steam and made remarkable contributions. Through his studies on bacterial genetics he developed an early basis for genetic engineering. Some of his contributions are now used in modern genetic engineering.

He predicted the increasing protein requirement of mankind and pondered whether it might not be better to abandon the sole emphasis on agriculture and, instead, cover this requirement more rapidly, more cheaply and better by the cultivation of protein-producing bacteria. He force-fed bacteria with amino acids, the building blocks of protein, while at the same time increasing the mutation rate (i.e. the tendency toward genetic change) by means of ultraviolet radiation and the addition of colchicine – the cell-altering chemical from the meadow saffron. This treatment killed most of the bacteria, since only a few could tolerate such high protein concentrations. These protein-tolerant bacteria were isolated and subjected to the same procedure once again. The repeated selection of protein-tolerant bacteria finally led to a strain of bacteria whose dry weight consisted of up to 85% protein and which was so used to the presence of proteins that it craved them and, when access to protein was reduced, produced it self-sufficiently from nitrogen, salts and cellulose. In the course of this procedure, the bacteria grew rapidly and multiplied enthusiastically.

Professor Wolf's process, the use of bacteria to produce protein for human consumption, was patented. Wolf presented the patent to Gandhi and President Roosevelt, and it is still lying somewhere in a patent archive.

These not exactly cheap investigations had been financed by his friend, the then Vice-President of the United States, Henry A. Wallace, who was actually a biologist and geneticist, and had, among other things, bred improved strains of wheat and larger strawberries.

More as a joke than anything else, Wolf created the world's first 'blue rose' for Vice-President Wallace via genetic manipulation. What was more important was that Wolf was able to grow immunizing bacteria by the same means for the successful fight against the udder inflammation of dairy cattle which was then reaching epidemic proportions in the United States.

During his intensive work in genetics, Wolf was becoming ever more conscious of the key role played by enzymes in everyday life and every living process. As he came to appreciate the enormous possibilities that lay in a mastery over the enzyme processes going on within the body, he limited his previously widespread interests and began to concentrate on enzyme research.

What is the *normal substance*?

It was for this reason that he got in touch with the Viennese physician Professor Dr. Ernst Freund. A report which appeared almost fantastic had reached the ears of the world in the early 1930's. Professor Freund and his coworker Dr. Kaminer had discovered that the blood of healthy people contained a substance which was capable of attacking and destroying cancer cells and thus acted as a defense against cancer. In the blood of patients suffering from cancer, this substance is either absent or only present to a slight degree. Professor Freund named this substance 'normal substance' without being able to say what this normal substance consisted of, or how it might work.

After the war, Wolf regularly travelled to Europe by ocean liner in order to exchange information with his European colleagues. It was during these exchanges that Wolf also informed himself about modern X-ray and radiation therapy against cancer and introduced it into America.

He was absolutely fascinated by the *'normal substance'* of Professor Freund. When Professor Freund died, he took over further research on the normal substance and soon concluded, quite correctly, that it could only be an enzyme.

He discovered that this substance which is normally present in the healthy, but absent or only present in small quantities in cancer patients, is a member of the hydrolase family of enzymes and requires a coenzyme for its activation.

He then investigated the hydrolases more closely and was able to show that when they falter they play an important role in the occurrence of cancer, and that the type, amount and quality of these enzymes is of primary importance to all health disturbances.

From this, Max Wolf drew the logical conclusion that the administration of the correct type, quantity and quality of hydrolases would be a fundamental medical measure for the restoration and guarantee of health, and could revolutionize the entire medical field.

The Biological Research Institute of New York

Professor Max Wolf founded the "Biological Research Institute" in New York and persuaded Dr. Helen Benitez, for many years head of the laboratory for cell culture techniques at the neurosurgical department of Columbia University, to work with him.

The first task of this biochemist was to isolate hydrolases from animal and vegetable sources and to free them from what may be termed 'foreign' proteins, regardless of the fact that hydrolases themselves are theoretically 'foreign' proteins. Enzymes are indeed very fussy concerning the substrates they capture and what they do with them, but whether they do it in an animal, a plant, a human being or a microorganism leaves them quite cold. Happily they are not species-specific, otherwise it would be impossible for us to take up a single enzyme from our food and utilize it in our bodies. Enzyme therapy in its entirety would be practically impossible.

Thousands of tests were then performed with the purified hydrolases. The question was which of the hydrolases from what animal, vegetable or microbial source possessed which activities.

In the laboratory, different concentrations of the hydrolases were added to cell cultures containing cancer cells. The suitability of the individual enzymes was measured in their ability to break down the cancer cells. An endless series of time-consuming experiments was used to select the most likely candidates from the vast number of available hydrolases.

These were then unified to mixtures which appeared optimal, taking care that the activity of each enzyme complemented that of the others, in order to achieve a broad spectrum of desired reactions.

After a number of years, three enzyme mixtures stood out, one appearing to be more effective on inflammatory, the second more on degenerative disorders and the third on cancer. These combinations of enzymes of animal and plant origin developed in the "Biological Research Institute" were named 'Wolf-Benitez enzyme mixtures'. However, a great deal of work had to be carried out before these enzyme mixtures could be offered throughout the world as drugs.

It was necessary to solve the problems of packing the enzymes into solid tablets, the optimal method of uptake into the body had to be determined and it had to be established that enzymes taken in a natural manner were harmless.

In order to achieve this, Professor Wolf fed incredibly high doses of his enzyme mixtures to animals. He wanted to be sure that such large quantities of enzymes did not get out of control and perhaps attack and break down the organism to which they were fed. Fortunately nothing bad happened. The enzymes only did what was required of them and did not run wild.

Since then, further experiments have been carried out again and again in order to uncover possible risks and to be sure that even the human body does not adapt in some way and perhaps stop making its own enzymes during long-term administration. Professor Haubold a well-known physician and scientist from Germany with a career that had been very succesful although not quite so spectacular as that of Max Wolf, continued this line of research with other European associates. At the time, Haubold was intensively involved in the investigation of vitamins and was working with his associates on the relationship between vitamin A deficiencies and certain diseases, particularly poliomyelitis.

Although treatment with vitamin A at high levels was required, the problem was to introduce it into the body in such a way as to minimize the side effects. The researchers managed this with a vitamin A emulsion that was absorbed in the same manner as mother's milk by an infant. This was accomplished, for the first time ever, by creating an emulsion composed of liposomes.

The problems of safe administration of the vitamin on the one hand, and of safe administration of enzymes on the other, complemented one another ideally. Aside from that, there were many other similarities. The scientists recognized the dimensions of this fascinating field and decided henceforth to dedicate their careers to enzymes and vitamin emulsions. Thus, they were able to develop a technology for stable encapsulation of enzymes which then were combined in the proper mixtures and converted to enteric-coated tablets to prevent their premature destruction by stomach acids when taken orally. The tablets then dissolved in the small intestine and their early research confirmed absorption.

Together with Professor Wolf, they founded the still existent "Medical Enzyme Research Institute", dedicated to the research and advancement of enzymes.

Artists, politicians, billionaires, stars

Professor Wolf had, in fact, treated many of his patients with enzyme mixtures from the start, with complete faith in their safety and efficacy. His efforts were crowned with success.

His patients included extremely wealthy and very famous persons. They were given these drugs which seemed so mysterious to other physicians and which were initially only manufactured in limited quantities. Although he would have wanted otherwise, they could not be made generally available. The drugs acquired the reputation of only being for the rich and famous of this world.

The fact that Professor Wolf became the elite personal physician of high society, although he cared little for the glitter and glamour of worldly life, was mainly due to a not very talented lady pianist who played in the orchestra of the Metropolitan Opera during the 1920's and one day suffered a traffic accident in which she was injured slightly. She was brought to the practice of the nearest physician; it happened to be the ENT practice of Professor Wolf.

He treated the lady pianist, but she was unable to pay his fee. At her request, she acted as his receptionist. Her name was Edith and she was very alert, very smart, and very fond of the good things in life. She realized what a genius Max Wolf was and how successful he was as a doctor, but how helpless he was in everyday practicalities. In her energetic way, she decided to look after everything and married him.

All went well for a while but one day she took out an advertisement in the New York Times without his knowledge. The advertisement claimed, "We guarantee the health of you and your family for $1,000 a year. Professor Dr. Max Wolf."

Professor Wolf had to resign his professorial chair after this enormous breach of professional ethics. He took the next ship to Europe and returned to Vienna without his somewhat impetuous wife Edith; there he abandoned medicine and once again took up painting.

His wife Edith was absolutely astonished by the whole furor. She still thought that the advertisement was a good idea. After the abrupt departure of her husband Max she felt destitute and followed a wealthy, young, good-looking admirer to Venice in order to amuse herself and have a good time with him there. Unfortunately, the wealthy, good-looking young man soon turned out to be not very amusing, but rather to be a crashing bore.

She walked out on him at the Lido in Venice and travelled on to Vienna, found her husband and persuaded him that he could not just give in; must not throw in the towel, but had to fight on. He therefore hung up his artist's smock, put on his white coat once again and returned to New York where the medical community graciously restored him to favor as well as restoring his professorship.

However, his wife Edith's unusual advertising methods were not without effect. Ever more famous people sought him out. The first artists to come to him became aware of him through his wife. She painted the great skills of her little Max in brilliant colors at the Metropolitan Opera. The musicians, singers, and conductors of the Met came to consult him, at first out of curiosity and then with enthusiasm. The enthusiasm for him eventually became so great that he was appointed official physician to the Met. Wolf, who was attracted by both music and medicine to the same degree, occupied the post with great delight for many years.

"Max Wolf and His Enzymes", the biography of this remarkable physician, is quite revealing about the life of this interesting man, details of his medical practice, his research and fascinating vignettes about the famous people whom he treated. The interested reader is referred to this book to learn more about this dynamo of a man. Here, one learns about the many rich and famous of the time that he treated. According to his biography, many celebrities from Hollywood and international personalities consulted him, as did many talented artists and musicians. He became very famous among the international politicians, the wealthy, the powerful and the personalities of the art world.

One learns in Dr. Wolf's biography that, "the tradition of taking these energizing novel medications to try to ensure good health has remained popular to this day in the artistic world, and that in our theaters, opera houses, film and television studios there are performing artists who repeatedly turn to oral enzyme tablets when not feeling well, or who have been taking them day in, day out for years, as a precautionary measure."

Wolf's biography detailed countless reports regarding many of the rich and the powerful personalities from the United States, Europe and other countries regularly consulting him, including presidents and high ranking government functionaries. He was the physician of the members of the great and wealthy families of America. Everywhere Professor Wolf went, the local establishment appeared. He was visited by prime ministers, dukes, famous writers, as well as by many disabled and terminally ill persons.

The end and a beginning

On the typewriter, he once wrote a manuscript, without periods or commas, but packed with anecdotes and scientific bonbons by the thousand; at the time, his as yet unpublished memoirs. He wrote at the end that he wanted to live to be a hundred.

That was perhaps the only unfulfilled ambition of Max Wolf, for he died at the age of 91. He was active to the end of his life, mentally alert, constantly planning for the future, very difficult and impatient, very lovable and helpful, knowledgeable, instructing and learning until the very end.

He was found to be suffering from stomach cancer in 1976. Too late and advanced when discovered, his colleagues gave his case up as inoperable. He was flown to Bonn at his own wish. There, in a clinic specializing in cancer, he was injected with enzymes, including some injections directly into the tumor site. The gastric tumor was thereby attacked by the hydrolases and began to dissolve. However, he appeared to be improving dramatically when renal failure subsequently developed. Professor Max Wolf died with a slight smile on his lips.

There was, in fact, a danger that enzyme therapy would die with Max Wolf. One could say that Wolf himself was the best enzyme for bringing about positive changes in the medical profession.

It is stated at the conclusion of his biography that for these reasons other scientists took on a great load with the scientific inheritance of Professor Wolf's work. They had two very difficult tasks. One was bringing a drug onto the market which was difficult and correspondingly expensive to manufacture, a product in need of constant quality improvements and demanded in ever increasing quantities. They also had to combat the skeptics, lack of understanding and even animosity of the specialist medical world. In addition, they had to demonstrate and reconfirm what Wolf had only been able to indicate in outline, namely that he had clinically studied these drugs in great detail and verified that they are safe to administer, do not cause any notable side effects, are compatible with other drugs, can be applied universally and that they actually bring about the health-promoting changes in the human body which are claimed of them.

It was necessary to demonstrate that this was no utopia, and yet that the negative and prevailing medical dogma could not deflate the dream of being able to administer the enzymes which they called the 'givers of health' to those who really needed them. Publications detailing the results of the work performed by Professor Wolf's disciples and coworkers afterwards indicate to a large extent that there is scientific documentation confirming their effectiveness and safety, and that the products are widely accepted in Europe and other countries. The dream of Max Wolf gradually has come true.

Chapter 8

Remedies: Efficacious and safe

How effective and safe can these preparations be? Regardless of the results, the issue is surrounded by controversy from its inception. It begins with the people running the health authorities of every country. One thing they are all in agreement with, whether they be from the FDA in the United States, the BGA in Germany or the authorities elsewhere – they all throw up their hands in horror as soon as they read the list of ingredients of the enzyme mixtures of Wolf and Benitez! It contains enzymes from animal origins, such as *pancreatin, chymotrypsin, trypsin, amylase and lipase*, and such plant enzymes as *papain and bromelain*, together with a little vitamin P (*rutin, a bioflavonoid*) or, in another mixture, *calves' thymus hydrolysates* and other *proteases*. On a first impression it appears to be an unlikely combination. The enzymes in the food which we consume during a meal also are unlikely combinations, and yet they help us.

Compound preparations! Laboratories are unable to compile reliable reports about them, what their contents are, what effects they produce, whether they mutually interfere with each other or what actually goes on.

One requirement from the authorities is that of order. Only one active component per drug, so that the function of this active agent can be precisely investigated. This demand is echoed by industrious preachers for improved pharmacology, as well as by the authors of publications which have taken a somewhat biased view.

If we strictly followed this advice without change, we would have to stop eating bread or drinking water. These are combination preparations whose compositions have not even been standardized and where the synergy of their components has not been exactly defined. In pharmacology, synergy is defined as the mutual support of several drugs or their components to one another's effects. From a pharmacological viewpoint, bread and water ought to be utterly rejected or only made available on prescription, with warning lists as long as your arm on the package inserts.

According to some scientists, "the entire history of the condemnation of combination preparations is truly an idea born in the misty realms of colorless theory, without a basis in the practical understanding of biochemical laws. The fact that some combination preparations are rather mischievous does not mean, by far, that all combination preparations are dubious drugs, to be banned from the pharmacy shelves."

The scientists point out that, in the case of the enzyme preparations which concern us here, there is, happily, sufficient evidence that combinations of enzymes were developed over a prolonged period of time through carefully designed scientific studies and through thousands of time consuming experiments, following the strict rules of scientific research and scientific principles. They were not merely chosen at random according to the motto "a little bit of everything and something will certainly help."

Correctly combined?

Every enzyme is a specialist, accepting only a certain substrate and changing this substrate only in a specific manner. They are only properly active in media of a certain acid or alkaline environment. If there is a disturbance in health, the situation is like that of a house on fire and it is not very helpful to merely run out a fire hose or to bring a ladder. Many things are required and they must interact with one another. If one person is missing from the bucket brigade, the fire cannot be put out.

Thus, it is necessary to make as wide a range of enzymes as possible available to the body so that no gaps of this kind arise.

According to enzyme scientists, the fact that the body is helped far better and more rapidly when different enzymes change various parts of the substrate at the same time is a further reason for the combination of enzymes. It must not be imagined that a substrate completely disappears into the active site of an enzyme, since only a tiny portion of the substrate will fit. There are gigantic substrates too that can be acted upon and cleaved by numerous enzymes at once (Figure 20). This can be compared to countless crustaceans the size of the palm of your hand attacking an aircraft carrier and sinking it via corrosion.

According to the scientists, another advantage of enzyme combinations lies, in part, in the fact that they contain enzymes of the same type but of different origins. In this way, it is possible to compensate for differing activities which can result with enzymes from the same source.

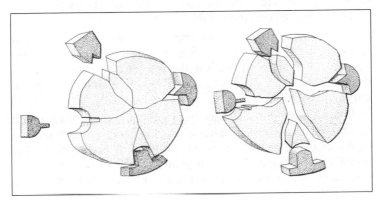

Figure 20: Various enzymes cleave a large substrate

Finally, according to them, there is a somewhat simpler example of the advantages of balanced enzyme combinations. Namely, their *synergism*. This results in greater and broader activity in practical application, as compared with single-enzyme preparations. The latter have only one enzyme as an active component. The activity of the total mixture is superior to any of the individual components.

One should remember that there are several single-enzyme preparations which can be administered orally as well, and which have a limited effect against some diseases or digestive disorders. The most famous is the enzyme product *Aniflazym* which has the largest worldwide sales by far. It contains the enzyme *serrapeptase* isolated from a microorganism that lives in the gut of the silkworm. The preparation is manufactured by the Takeda company and is one of the drugs taken most frequently in Japan. Other single-enzyme products contain *pancreatin* obtained from the pancreas, *papain* from papayas or *bromelain* from pineapples.

They can all be used effectively in particular circumstances, although single-enzyme preparations have not been demonstrated to produce as wide-ranging and distinct effects as has been reported with the enzyme combinations.

At any rate, most single-enzyme preparations are, strictly speaking, small scale combination preparations. *Pancreatin*, for instance, does not contain just the one enzyme, but at least a dozen. *Papain* and *bromelain* are also combinations of several enzymes.

Enough said, the scientists have gradually made their point; that the relatively large number of varying components combined in the enzyme mixtures appears not to be a disadvantage, but rather an advantage. They also point out that it is also another reason for the unique and remarkable effect of the drug in so many different fields.

A question of safety

None of this, however, answers the question as to whether the enzyme mixtures could possibly be dangerous, whether there is a risk of the foreign enzymes ganging up against us, going mad and breaking us down into our individual components. Of course, the question of the drug's safety is particularly important since, according to the claimed indications and usage, such enzyme combinations can, under certain circumstances, be taken over long periods of time and at relatively high doses.

Some questions to be answered are as follows, "When do the enzymes that are administered begin to be harmful or even poisonous?," "What side effects can they bring about?," "How do they alter the fetus during pregnancy?" and "Do they perhaps alter cells?"

Results of the published studies on these subjects are illuminating. These drugs have been fed to numerous laboratory animals in a dose one hundredfold larger than that advocated for humans. The latter included guinea pigs, rats, rabbits and dogs. Before animal lovers rush to the barricades, let us add quickly that the animals were scarcely affected. All that happened was that some of them temporarily demonstrated changes in their appetites and tempers.

It was impossible to determine the lethal dose since the animals survived outrageously large quantities without damage. Guinea pigs and rats, for example, were fed a daily dose of enzyme mixtures for six months which would have corresponded to approximately 250 tablets per day for a 60 kg man. The animals demonstrated no negative effects whatsoever. Female rats were fed a dose corresponding to a human dose of 2,500 tablets daily for a short period and their organs gained a little in weight and they appeared somewhat fatigued.

Mutations, i.e. cell changes, were not found to occur after enzyme mixture administration. The enzymes found in the mixture were added to cell cultures and a search was made for evidence of cell toxicity or mutation. No harmful changes were found, the enzyme preparations proved to be safe.

Not for everyone: The contraindications

There are of course limitations to all drugs. Animal experiments are not necessary to establish this. According to the European scientists, "care should be taken with enzyme preparations during pregnancy since it is a rule to be careful with drugs in general when expecting. Even though the new life in the womb is only likely to be affected by extremely high doses of enzymes, it is probably better not to even take a theoretical risk. Likewise, nursing mothers should avoid taking enzymes since these could affect the milk."

The scientists also declare that, "the second contraindication for taking enzyme preparations concerns hemophiliacs and other patients whose blood is so thin that blood coagulation does not set in and the danger of bleeding exists with every small injury. Here, blood-flow equilibrium is so disturbed that the enzyme mixtures could further inactivate blood coagulants, one of their known functions. This could amplify the disorder since their antagonists are lacking. Enzyme preparations should not be taken shortly before or after surgical intervention involving a high risk of bleeding either, so that a control of hemorrhage is not affected adversely. They are not recommended for patients on 'blood thinners'. The blood of patients taking anticoagulant preparations also lacks antagonists and enzyme preparations could enhance the liquefaction of the blood too much."

Interactions and side effects

Apart from the case of concomitant anticoagulant therapy, the scientists point out that the interactions of enzymes with other drugs are a further plus in their favor. They emphasize, for instance, that, "it has been established that equivalent doses of chemotherapeutic drugs have greater effects when taken together with enzyme mixtures." They claim that, "this also applies to antibiotics, including sulfonamides, steroid preparations (cortisone) and cytostatics (anticancer agents)", and that, "All of these represent drugs with a substantial risk of side effects." They reported that, "scientific investigations demonstrating that the enzyme mixtures are able to increase the effect of eleven extremely problematic chemotherapeutic agents by from 8 to 40%." This was interpreted to mean that, "in order to obtain the effect desired by the physician, the dose and, hence, the risks can be reduced to this degree. The effects of other drugs were increased and their side effects reduced when administered together with the enzyme mixtures."

The interactions can be regarded as positive, but what about the side effects?

According to the scientists, "some people, estimated to be 50% of those taking enzymes, reveal a harmless change in the nature, color and odor of their stools. The odor is reminiscent of the scent of tomcats. This may be considered a nuisance, but it is of no importance and usually disappears within a few days. These effects are caused by activated enzymes which do not proceed into the bloodstream and lymph tract, but instead follow the normal pathway through the bowels."

Generally, tablets containing the enzyme mixtures are candy coated. That is because the enzymes in the mixtures do not smell too pleasant either. The taste of the actual enzymes is also somewhat unpleasant as can be confirmed by anyone who has mistaken the coated tablets for candies and chewed one.

Doesn't anything else happen? Multiple enzyme mixture preparations are available worldwide. The three enzymatic preparations containing mixtures developed by Wolf and Benitez have been available commercially in Europe since 1976 and have been prescribed more than 20 million times. Unprescribed administration is substantially higher since one of the preparations is available over-the-counter as a 'digestive' in some countries.

A total of about 240 cases of side effects have been reported. These were predominantly complaints due to increased gas formation in the bowels or slightly increased bleeding tendencies following surgery or injury. There were rare cases of slight burning or itching of the skin after enemas containing enzymes. Allergic reactions were limited to injectable preparations or enemas and occurred very rarely (see introduction).

The scientists indicated that presumed anaphylactoid reactions to foreign proteins were only recorded in three cases. "So", the skeptics will say, "as we thought!" Further, they will say "These highly-praised and supposedly harmless enzyme preparations which can be taken over-the-counter can indeed cause the same anaphylactic reactions known from the infusion of streptokinase, urokinase and other preparations. Such preparations must be applied with utmost care and, if at all, only by hospital physicians."

According to the European scientists, "Anaphylactoid reactions only occurred when enzyme preparations were combined with the local anesthetics procaine or lidocaine, added to reduce the pain of the injection. As every dentist knows, procaine or lidocaine, with their protein content, can occasionally lead to anaphylactic reactions." They further stated that, "the three cases reported cannot be attributed to enzymes since the patients subsequently had more enzymes without problems. Most likely they were due to the anesthetic or one of its inert components, such as the preservatives." Some forms and dosages of anesthetic are still manufactured containing methyl-paraben and sodium metabisulfite as preservatives. These are known to produce allergic reactions in some individuals.

Thus, neither during pregnancy, nor when breast-feeding, not for hemophiliacs, nor directly pre or postoperative to surgery with an increased risk of hemorrhage, and what else? Stool can become pale or smell like a tomcat, microenemas can sometimes cause the perianal area to itch or burn.

Some will caution that, since there are some side effects, the harmlessness of these medications does not seem to stand the test, or does it? Just read the long list of contraindications, adverse effects, concomitant symptoms, interactions, notifications and warnings for any drugs said to be safe. "It will then be clear that there are scarcely any drugs as harmless as such enzyme preparations."

Some physicians who do not believe in the effectivity of enzyme preparations have emphasized this harmlessness in their arguments. They say, "Drugs which are so harmless and cause so few side effects cannot be so effective either, since there are no effects without side effects." In other words, and according to these physicians, the more side effects, the better the efficacy and, therefore, the better the drug! Apparently only dangerous drugs with a plethora of side effects should be put on the market.

The point is, what is absorbed?

Review of the data published by the European scientists appeared most interesting and illuminating. In this section, we will review their arguments and responses to criticisms voiced by other more traditional medical practitioners. The argument concerning lack of effect is by far the most important weapon relied on by opponents of 'systemic' oral enzyme therapy. Here, they feel they may have found a tool to completely remove what they believe to be a scientifically utterly unjustifiable method from the medical agenda.

We have therefore saved the most frequent argument until the end for more detailed consideration. The situation is crystal clear, if the enzymes really cannot pass from the intestinal tract into the circulatory lymphatic systems and thereby reach other parts of the organism to unfold their purported pharmacological and healing effects by their very presence, we better forget the whole thing.

There is one argument for the efficacy of enzyme preparations that is convincing, but it sounds somewhat confusing. If such drugs such as the anti-inflammatory enzyme mixtures are taken for an inflammatory disease, the patient frequently notices that the inflammation becomes more intense. The whys and wherefores of the reasons for regarding this as a favorable sign for beginning recovery will be explained in more detail in the chapter on inflammation. In the opinion of the European scientists, this represents what is described as an *initial deterioration* that is soon alleviated and leaves the way open for recovery.

"It is not a side effect, it is an effect", but a demonstration of this type will certainly not convince skeptics. Scientists wish to know and wish to see publications, laboratory results, tests, graphs and statistics. They demand a demonstration of the presence of the foreign enzyme in the circulation and in the entire human organism after it has been taken in by the natural route, to demonstrate absorption.

The skeptics point their fingers at the textbooks which earnestly maintain that such macromolecules as enzymes are unable to pass the barrier of the intestinal wall and thereby cannot reach the bloodstream and lymph tract.

What actually are macromolecules? A compound made up of two or more atoms is known as a molecule. When more than 1,000 atoms are bonded together in one molecule, this is known as a macromolecule. The enzyme preparations entering the organism via the natural route contain nothing but enzymes and are rather large macromolecules. Their molecular structures range from between 18,000 and 60,000 atoms per molecule.

That the textbooks cannot be completely right can be seen from two facts. First, macromolecules such as bile and pancreatic enzymes have been shown to be reabsorbed back into the circulation from the intestine where they are released by the pancreas. This is known as the enterobiliary and enteropancreatic circulation. Another example of absorption of macromolecules occurs in nursing babies, born without any protection against bacterial infection, who take up the antibodies from the mother's milk, providing them with the necessary protection, and that these antibodies pass from the intestines into the circulatory and lymphatic systems and thereby permeate the baby's entire body. Antibodies are also macromolecules with a size comparable to that of the enzymes. These antibodies are also known as gamma globulins.

In order to investigate the absorption of such macromolecules more carefully, Professor Seifert of the University Surgical Clinic in Kiel labeled horse gammaglobulins radioactively and fed them by mouth to rats and dogs; humans took them as well. These equine gamma globulins are extremely large and have a molecular weight of 120,000.

The researcher reported that they were absorbed. This means they were taken up from the intestines and their presence was demonstrable throughout the bodies of dogs, rats and humans.

This contradicted the next argument helpfully drawn upon by opponents, namely, that foreign macromolecules such as enzymes entering the stomach and intestines can only act as a sort of a fuse to stimulate the production of similar intrinsic enzymes (inherent to the body) throughout the whole body. A signal, nothing more.

However, the critics were not self-conscious and soon found another argument. It is quite clear, they said, that these foreign molecules enter the blood and lymph because they are cleaved enzymatically in the intestinal tract and then transported through the narrow intestinal villi as tiny fragments and can thereby enter the bloodstream and lymph tract.

Professor Seifert undertook further experiments and proved unequivocally, by means of immunological testing systems, that the gamma globulins were not broken down, but entered the rest of the body unaffected and in full size.

The counterarguments continued to become ever more threadbare. The one used now is as follows, "Very good, perhaps gamma globulins or other antibodies can be absorbed, but enzymes most certainly cannot." This argument has also been addressed by Seifert and other scientists. The enzyme scientists allege that more and more investigations on the absorption of macromolecules from the intestinal tract into the rest of the body carried out in many universities and hospitals have finally laid this old dogma to rest.

It is now known that uptake of large molecules into the whole organism is certainly dependent on the size of the molecule but, nevertheless, that some very large macromolecules are even absorbed better than some smaller ones. In the case of enzymes, it has been reported that their absorption depends on their origin, on their concentration and activity, on the milieu of the intestinal tract and on other individual prerequisites.

According to published reports, numerous test methods for determination of the absorption rate, i.e. the determination of how much enzyme appears within the body, support the concept that this absorption takes place. However, they have not yielded uniform results concerning the amounts absorbed, since they all use somewhat different measurement techniques. This restriction applies to all macromolecules and not only to enzymes.

The studies purport that, "it has thereby been scientifically demonstrated that such macromolecules as the individual enzymes found in the anti-inflammatory enzyme mixtures can pass undamaged through the intestinal wall and further into the whole organism." However, on account of the differing methods of measurement, there is no agreement as to what percentage of the enzyme taken actually makes the successful journey into the body without being damaged.

To the journey's end

Of course, not every enzyme taken by mouth, applied to the skin or introduced in the form of a microenema reaches the site in the body where it is urgently required, 'full of beans' and undamaged. The enzyme army suffers grievous losses en route. Only the strongest, the toughest or the luckiest enzymes reach their goal in an active state. That is why, based on the experiences in Europe, a larger number of oral tablets are required to obtain the desired therapeutic responses. Contrary to the customary oral dosages of 1 to 4 or 5 tablets daily used in other fields of medicine, the oral enzymes have to be given in dosages of up to 20 or more tablets daily, given in divided dosages of 4 or 5 tablets several times daily. This is, in part, because only a portion of the oral dosage is felt to be absorbed and, in part, due to other factors which will be discussed below.

It was long believed that enzymes taken as tablets or pills would be broken down in the stomach. According to Wolf and Benitez, some of the enzyme preparations are treated to make them resistant to gastric juices and have a protective coat which does not dissolve until the preparation reaches the intestines. Furthermore, it has since been shown that the enzyme preparations are not attacked by the gastric juices to the extent previously feared.

Scientists believe that some of the enzymes swallowed in the inactive state are activated in the intestinal tract. There, they can precipitate a bloated feeling and flatulence and cause changes in the condition, appearance and odor of the stool. Enzymes find their way into the intestines more directly when they are administered rectally, i.e. with the help of microenemas.

For a long time, it was a mystery how macromolecules managed to make the journey through or between the narrow intestinal villi into the circulatory and lymphatic systems. The macromolecules actually appear to use three ingenious methods for overcoming this barrier. It would be going too far here to indulge in long, complicated explanations of the mechanism of transport, but it takes place in a manner similar to the return of unused pancreatic juices from the intestinal tract into the circulation. It is generally accepted in medicine that the healthy pancreas produces relatively large quantities of pancreatic fluid containing *pancreatin* and other enzymes, and that not all of it is used. Reabsorption of the unused portion has been termed the *enteropancreatic circulation*. Thrifty as nature is, it always collects this unused juice and returns it to the pancreas. It does so by transferring it from the intestinal tract to the circulatory system and then back into the pancreas. A quite remarkable little circulation which leads a Cinderella existence as far as medicine is concerned, but which is worthy of more attention.

No matter how brilliant the method may be by which the enzymes cross the barrier of the intestinal villi and enter the circu-

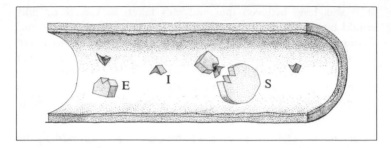

Figure 21: Enzyme inhibitors (I) interact with enzymes in the bloodstream

latory and lymphatic systems, the journey is a difficult undertaking, involving losses as far as enzymes are concerned.

The reduced forces compared with the amounts of enzymes taken originally will interact in the blood with the body's own protease inhibitors (Figure 21). These protein inhibitors, the most important of which seems to be alpha-2 macroglobulin (α-2M), are transport and regulatory molecules of the immune system. These α–2Ms transport cell messenger substances (cytokines) through the tissue and regulate their function. One of these cytokines, the tumor necrosis factor (TNF) acts as a weapon against tumor-cells. The effect of orally administered proteolytic enzymes is regulated by the α–2Ms. Additionally, α-2M covers those parts of the enzyme molecule which could lead to an allergic reaction. This α-2M is formed in the monocytes and macrophages and is also eliminated by these cells.

The enzyme researchers indicate that when you realize the difficulties and heavy casualties involved in the journey of the poor enzymes before they can finally perform their activities, you begin to understand why so many tablets are usually prescribed and why it is not very helpful to swallow just one tablet each day.

Another point they make is that it is also best to take the enzyme preparations on an empty stomach. When you are fasting the other enzymes of the stomach and intestinal tract are not fully active so that more troops can get through without losses.

They suggest that the anti-inflammatory enzyme mixtures should also be taken several times daily, at least mornings and evenings, since, after activation (by water and oxygen), the hydrolases contained in the enzyme mixtures are only active in the body for a maximum of five hours.

Taking many tablets several times daily is only possible when it is known that the drugs will not result in serious damage. Again, the scientists emphasize, according to the published reports, that it is fortunate that the enzymes are quite safe, so that even extremely large doses do not cause serious damage. The reason for this remarkable margin of safety is because of the fact that only a certain percentage of the enzymes are available to the organism in an active state. How much is that? One enzyme in a hundred? The results of all the scientific investigations thus far available point to an absorption rate of 12-20%, so that one fifth of the oral dosage of hydrolases taken can be available to exert their activity where they are required within the body. With a newer mixture, up to ~40% absorption has been reported.

The question of the proportion absorbed is not very important if the amount absorbed actually works. However, it may be of importance to the biochemist. Not even the lawmakers are very interested in the amount absorbed. The 'guidelines for drug examination of 1986' state, in that impressive language of the lawmaker, "Since methods are not available for the measurement of substance concentration, the time-response curves of a reliably measurable pharmacodynamic effect of the substance (effect kinetics) can be accepted."

Stated more simply, "It is not necessary to determine how much substance is required to bring about a particular effect, as long as the effect itself can be demonstrated and measured."

The fact that the scientists are convinced enzymes work has, we hope, by now become clear. If so, the next question is how they work and what they work against. Also, what health disorders can be treated and improved by taking enzmyes via the oral route. The European experience suggests that the enzymes have a beneficial therapeutic effect on various disturbances affecting the body's defense system, including inflammations, injuries, circulatory disturbances, cell degeneration and viral infections. The enzymes also have been used preventively to minimize the ill effects associated with the gradually sinking enzyme activity of the body during aging. All of these conditions have one common denominator. Inflammation occurs, fibrin deposits at the sites of inflammation, the body defenses are called to repair the conflict, immune complexes develop, and fibrin is deposited further around these immune complexes and associated defense agents. Abortive attempts of our defenses to eliminate the blocking cascade of changes unfortunately result in tissue damage that causes more damage and leads to many of the degenerative diseases, cancer and other health disorders of mankind. According to the scientists, enzymes then help eliminate the excessive fibrin and to break down the excessive immune complexes,thus allowing our own defenses to function more effectively and to better protect us.

Chapter 9

Powers of defense: The body more than the doctor

Is there a more important topic to our health than that of the body's own defenses? What about the major diseases, the treatment of which is of much more interest to us than a discussion of the immune system? The latter is responsible for our internal defenses, but it is so complicated that even physicians sometimes have difficulties in understanding all aspects of it.

Well, our defenses are of extreme importance. That is the reason we are starting with the topic of this remarkable system responsible for everything to do with health or sickness, with immunology, and with the possibility of reinforcing the body's defense systems so that it is able to maintain our health and heal us when we are sick.

Afterall, it is not medicine which 'cures', not the drug. No doctor can heal a wound. He or she can contribute toward its healing, can relieve the strain on the body in many ways, support it, but healing and maintenance of health is the responsibility of the body's own defenses.

Astonishingly, the words immune system were not part of the physician's vocabulary 40 years ago. In those days, one would have sought in vain in the medical dictionaries for details of the system that protects our body every second of its life, which constantly attacks and destroys such intruding enemies as bacteria and viruses, breaks down toxins and wastes, and transports them away and protects us from cancer. One would have searched in vain for indications of that most important system of all which should always be thought of first.

Today, it seems unthinkable to us that you could discuss the treatment of disease without including the body's defenses, detoxification or elimination. From colds to AIDS, there is, in all probability, not one illness that can be combated without considering immunology.

It is not easy to describe this branch of medicine. For one thing, the immune system is perhaps the most complicated organ system of all, with hundreds of control mechanisms, and for another, our understanding of this unbelievably complicated system is relatively new and by no means complete. Finally, there are problems in translating the specialist jargon used to describe these processes in scientific publications into something generally comprehensible.

Therefore, every attempt to describe the basic outlines of the body's endogenous defenses, or to explain what happens when the defenses break down, or themselves become a source of disease, twists to and fro between efforts to be factually correct and understandable. The reader should be prepared to take part in this slalom course because it will lead to something worthwhile. Knowledge concerning the principle that protects your very life and knowledge of how your life can be helped with these principles is of great importance to all of us.

Identify, catch and consume enemies

Strictly speaking, there is not only one immune system, but at least two. Let us start with the most general, with the 'nonspecific immune system' or 'sanitation department' of the body. Its primary means of detoxifying the body and carrying away the broken down by-products are the large, fat phagocytes that are hungry for all damaging matter.

They are known as macrophages, in English 'large eaters'. These macrophages, in their millions, permeate our entire body; they seek out, surround, take in, break down (we are back to our enzymes again), and spit out or transport away foreign bodies of all types (Figure 22). These include not only microorganisms penetrating from outside, but also external chemical toxins, the body's own wastes, dying, no longer functioning cells, early cancerous cells, and toxins produced by the body.

The detoxification and elimination of toxic materials of all types brought about by macrophages is naturally of extraordinary importance for the maintenance of health. It is to our advantage to lavish care and attention on our hungry macrophages, although this unfortunately seldom occurs. Numerous environmental toxins, stressful, unhealthy life styles, ranging from unsuitable diets to drug abuse, as well as many modern chemotherapeutic drugs, all can serve to inhibit these macrophages.

If macrophages are inhibited to any degree or for any length of time, more and more metabolic residues begin to accumulate in the blood, in the lymph and in the tissues which then lead to chronic illnesses.

This general, the *nonspecific defense system* with the omnivorous macrophages is accompanied and aided by the specific defense system for waste removal and detoxification.

Let us now look at the *specific defense system*. First of all, primitive stem cells are produced from bone marrow. These cells then differentiate into T-cells and B-cells (Figure 23). The T-cells get their special instructions in the thymus, hence the 'T', and the B-cells get their special instructions from ... well from somewhere. Perhaps in certain sections of the intestinal tract, in the spleen or somewhere else. We still do not know exactly where, except in the case of birds. They have a little pocket in their intestines, in Latin *bursa*, and this *bursa* gives us the 'B' for B-lymphocytes. However, a complete catalog distinguishing the whole range of T- and B-cells is of little help in a chapter on the use of enzymes for strengthening the immune system. Let us therefore concentrate on just one mechanism chosen from the whole story. B-cells are able to produce specific antibodies and to release these en masse into the circulatory and lymphatic systems to search for quite specific enemies. They can be compared to a tiny but powerful factory constantly producing antibodies on demand.

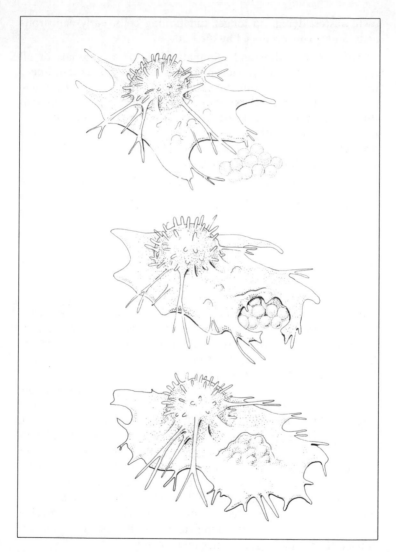

Figure 22: A macrophage "consumes" bacteria

An antibody is rather like a Y in shape. It has a long leg at the bottom and splits at the top end into two specially shaped claw arms. Using these arms, it untiringly feels the shapes of all the substances it comes into contact with. Almost all substances carry specific recognition signs or 'markers' on their exteriors. Should the claw arms fit the recognition signs, they then slip into place and remain attached (Figures 4, 5, 6 and 24). Antibodies only have claw arms for foreign substances, with a subtle mechanism making it possible for your body only to undertake cell-destroying measures when it is quite sure that it is directing them against foreign bodies. A wonderful system, although at times small errors result and serious consequences develop.

Such foreign cells as bacteria and viruses are recognized as being foreign, as so-called *antigens*, but chemicals or degenerate endogenous cells are also antigens. The degeneration into cancer cells causes what were previously worthy body cells to turn into malignant cancer cells with foreign labels or markers which could theoretically be recognized by antibodies and thereby arrested. When antibodies attach themselves to an antigen, an immune complex is formed (Figures 4, 5, 6 and 24). Every immune complex transmits signals indicating that other body defenses should come and destroy it. The immune complex thereby gives the command for its own execution.

The ever voracious macrophages are ideally suited to obey such commands. They are therefore pleased to appear, to engulf the immune complex and to break it down enzymatically.

However, all this is not sufficient for our bodies, better safe than sorry. The immune complex therefore alarms another death squad called the *complement system* as well. Complement is the somewhat confusing name given to a fantastic army of proteins containing at least nine principal components with multiple and different enzymes. They are, and this is easily forgotten, nothing more or less than another sort of our famous protein-degrading enzymes (Figure 1 and Figure 26).

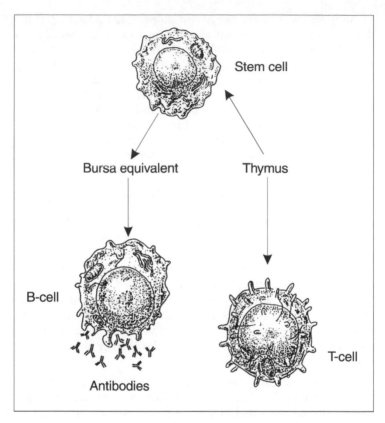

Figure 23: Formation of B- and T-cells

Basically, complement refers collectively to a group of plasma proteins and glycoproteins that constitute a powerful weapon in the body's defense system. They serve three major functions: The *first* is destruction by bursting ('lysis') of unwanted cells, such as early cancer cells, or lysis of bacteria, or of viruses having an envelope. The *second* function is the preparation of unwanted cellular

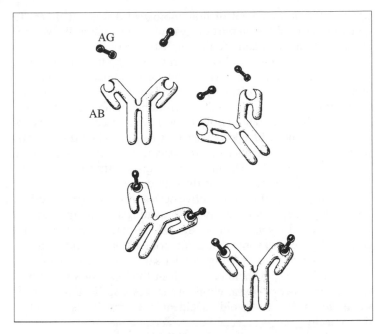

Figure 24: Antibodies (Ab) bind antigens (Ag)

debris or foreign particles (from bacteria, viruses, fungi, protozoans, etc.) for removal by the macrophages (phagocytosis). This is performed by coating the particles with the complement proteins which can be recognized by receptors in the phagocytic cells. The *third* function is regulation of inflammatory and immune responses. This is accomplished via 'mediators' which lead to migration of specific motile cells such as monocytes, release of histamine by degranulation of mast cells, activation of 'adhesion molecules', etc. The natural function of the complement is protective as a host defense. Unfortunately, excessive generation of the active fragments can lead to excessive inflammation, tissue damage and the development of immunological disease at times. To better understand this important system, let us look at the various steps involved, in an admittedly simplistic overview.

The immune complex always alarms only the first complement soldier in the system (Figures 26 and 1). This appears at the site, attaches itself to the antibody and calls for the second complement soldier. This goes on and on, with one member of the system activating the next. The whole thing is reminiscent of a row of upright dominoes which knock each other over when the first one falls. It is the last member of the system, the ninth complement, that is the actual killer. The immune complex is then destroyed, or the germ or cancer cell is lysed (broken down).

The purpose of this consecutive series of activations is safety. The body is determined to avoid activating that dangerous last killer at the wrong time, or in the wrong place, where it could conceivably destroy some living components of the body. Atomic warheads are also activated by similar safe-guarding systems. It is not possible to shoot them off merely at the touch of a single button, several interlocking preliminary stages also have to be activated in order to avoid accidents as much as possible, theoretically.

But theory is one thing, something can always go wrong in practice. Unfortunately, this is also true of the body's defenses and the breakdown of immune complexes. The activation of macrophages and the complement system depends, among other things, on the size and numbers of the immune complexes and also on whether they are floating freely in the bloodstream or lymph tract, or whether they have been deposited in the tissues. In other words, whether they are, *circulating* in the blood or what is called, *tissue-bound*.

Immune complexes are not all equal

In recent years, a special branch of immunology has emerged concerned with the question, "Which immune complexes trigger what signals; what inhibits and what promotes their degradation?"

Unfortunately, the formation of immune complexes is by no means as simple as 'one and one makes two'. Things do not normally proceed as they appear, that an antibody meets an antigen that fits, clings to it, shouts to alarm a killer, and after the kill the macrophage comes, gulps swiftly, and the immune complex is gone and digested.

Antibodies are usually tiny and the ill-intentioned foreign cells are very large. At first the antibodies only grasp hold with one of their arms and use the other one to clasp onto another foreign cell. A large aggregate of foreign cells and antibodies therefore results.

Sometimes the antibodies are present in excess, sometimes the ratio is about equal and sometimes the antigens dominate. What usually happens is that the antibody attaches itself to one or two antigens and this tiny immune complex floats freely around in the blood or the lymph. It is no longer dangerous and is frequently ingested by macrophages along the way, but it can also be overlooked because its signal is not really very strong.

Further antibodies then come into contact with the tiny immune complex and these, in turn, grasp further antigens, the immune complex grows. When it has reached a considerable size it then becomes a regular treat for a passing macrophage. Afterall, macrophages prefer such fat immune complexes and practically ignore everything else.

The moderately-sized immune complexes interest the macrophages least. If they do not grow by being coupled to more antibodies and more antigens, most moderately-sized immune complexes float around until they land somewhere on the tissue wall, penetrate this tissue and deposit themselves there. There they become *pathogenic immune complexes*. In the tissues, the macrophages are unable to reach them as easily. The available macrophages are usually less active anyway since, paradoxically, the greater the amount of immune complexes present in the body,

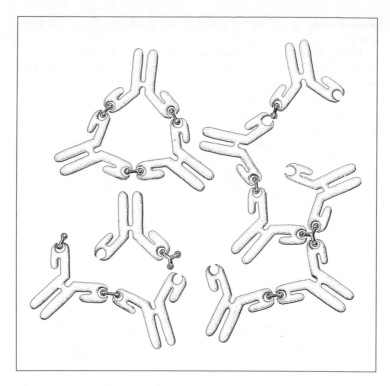

Figure 25:   Formation of immune complexes

the more the macrophages are inhibited in their activity. Instead of being able to deploy more and more hungry macrophages, the number of these hungry helpers in the organism diminishes just when they are needed most.

We destroy ourselves: Autoaggression

In this situation, the tissue-bound immune complexes activate the second defense system, the *complement system* (Figure 1 and

26). The death squad arrives, one enzyme after the other, the entire enzyme cascade is activated. An enormous protein-destroying activity is set in motion and brings about an inflammatory reaction. The result is tissue destruction. In many instances, this is the beginning of what is known as an autoaggressive or autoimmune disease, the organism attacks itself.

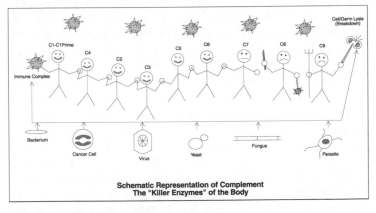

Figure 26: Complement cascade

Should such immune complexes collect in the tissues of the kidneys, for instance, complement activation can bring about inflammation that leads to glomerulonephritis (Figure 27). This process is now well-documented. There is little doubt of its existence. According to Wolf and Benitez, the enzyme preparations can prevent the glomerulonephritis as a result of enzymatic interruption of the complement cascade leading to killer activation.

Recent clinical studies published in Germany indicate that other immune complex disorders with similar origins can be treated in the same manner. Some of these are diseases which have been difficult or impossible to influence medically in the past. For instance, the studies report highly encouraging results in

Crohn's disease or ulcerative colitis, where the chronic intestinal inflammation is indirectly precipitated by the deposition of immune complexes in the intestinal tissue.

The proposed mechanism of action of enzymes in these disorders includes enzymatic interruption of the autoaggressive complement cascade, the enzymatic breakdown of pathogenic immune complexes and the important activation of the macrophages. They claim that, "this breaks the vicious cycle which otherwise leads to continual deterioration, thus making the disorder chronic, a never-ending circle of ever increasing immune complexes, which inhibit more macrophages, so that less immune complexes are broken down, so that more macrophages are inhibited, etc."

This vicious cycle of tissue injury due to immune complexes occurs in a number of diseases that can affect many organs. For example, the medical literature indicates that it can lead to pulmonary fibrosis in the lungs and to inflammation of the pancreas (chronic relapsing pancreatitis). The list of autoaggressive diseases caused by immune complexes is long. The type of disease does not only depend on the site where the immune complexes are immobilized, since freely circulating immune complexes can also lead to diseases of this type depending on their size and binding, or if substantial macrophage inhibition is present. Last but not least, a factor which plays a role is the source of the antigen.

Rheumatic diseases, e.g. rheumatoid arthritis or rheumatoid spondylitis, glomerulonephritis (a chronic inflammation of the kidney) and such inflammatory diseases of the intestinal tract as ulcerative colitis or Crohn's disease are typical autoaggressive diseases. Infection by certain viruses, bacteria and parasites are felt to also lead to autoaggressive diseases in some cases. Infectious hepatitis (jaundice) and shingles, for instance, are examples of diseases caused by viruses. Bacterial infections can cause such diseases as syphilis and may also cause heart muscle inflammations. Parasites cause malaria and toxoplasmosis. All diseases have an

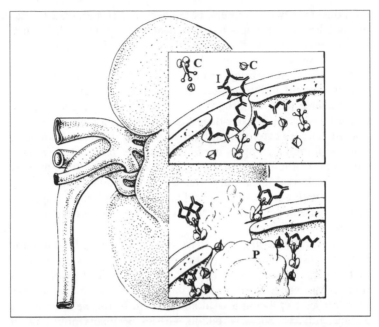

Figure 27: Schematic diagram of the development of glomerulonephritis. Enlarge-
ments show the fine structures of the renal tissue. Above: Immune complexes have formed in the tissue, complement (C) becomes activated.
Below: Complement activates the inflammatory process and incites the
mobility of macrophages, also known as phagocytes (P), to the site of
activity; destruction begins.

immune component based on the response of the body's defenses,
but not all lead to autoaggressive diseases.

What can be done?

Unfortunately, medicine is not very successful in the treatment
of autoimmune diseases. Hundreds of different treatments have
been used for these diseases with rather poor results. Since the

relationship between immune complexes and certain diseases has become known, attempts have been made to prevent the formation of immune complexes and to suppress the inflammations caused by the activity of complement.

For this purpose, drugs are used to weaken the activity of the immune system and to suppress the symptoms of inflammation.

If patients receive a drug that weakens the body's defenses, so-called immunosuppressive drugs, cortisone being among the best-known, but also cytotoxic (anticancer) drugs, the patient suffering from an immune complex-mediated disorder feels better initially since one of the effects of such drugs is to reduce the antibody concentrations. This means that fewer antibodies can actually combine with antigens in the body and yield immune complexes. Fewer immune complexes naturally lead to fewer effects caused by immune complexes.

However, in the long run, these medications may be doing the body an unintentional disservice in this way since, when used in high dosages or long enough, they weaken its defenses. In addition to various side effects, an immunosuppressed person can therefore end up being a weakened victim of the next attack by enemy antigens. Bacteria, bacilli, viruses or toxins now have it easier, and the risk of cancer is also appreciably increased when such drugs are taken for a long period.

The inflammation-inhibiting drugs frequently prescribed for immune complex-mediated diseases actually inhibit the inflammation because they interfere with the mechanism of inflammation. This causes, among other things, a reduction of pain frequently associated with the inflammation. Nevertheless, the defense squads (complement components) still continue to damage the organism and immune complexes are not eliminated. Inflammation inhibitors treat the symptoms, but not their causes.

A further alternative method appears more promising. Here, an attempt is made to remove the immune complexes from the blood before they have a chance to attach themselves to the tissue and cause their mischief. This consideration has led to the use of effective physical measures since it was discovered that kidney patients dependent on dialysis and also suffering from disease caused by immune complexes noticed an improvement in the symptoms of the immune complex-mediated disease after dialysis. It was thereby concluded that blood washing probably also filtered out pathogenic immune complexes.

There are several methods in which the blood can, as it were, be washed clean. The best method of removing immune complexes from the blood so far is the process known as *membrane plasmapheresis* (Figure 41). About 1 to 2 liters of blood are removed from the patient and, while outside the body, the solid part of the blood containing the cells is removed from the liquid part, the plasma. The plasma is then filtered through a special membrane which is able to stop and remove immune complexes and other proteins. The purified plasma is then combined with the solid portion of the blood and returned to the patient's circulatory system.

This plasmapheresis can save lives by removing toxins from the blood. It is very complicated and associated with some side effects (allergy, calcium deficiency, reduced blood pressure, fever, shivering, blood coagulation disturbances, etc.). It costs over $1,000 per treatment. Since it has to be repeated regularly for patients with immune response-mediated diseases, the whole thing becomes a question of money as well as of bodily stress and the risk of side effects.

For this reason, an attempt is made to make the interval between two plasmapheresis sessions as long as possible. In addition, the removal of the pathogenic substances acts as a stimulation for the formation of more pathogenic substances, a rebound effect which can result in the disorder progressing.

Nevertheless, plasmapheresis is an important measure to be recommended for a very acute and severe attack, in an emergency situation. An improvement is also to be expected in the case of chronic, immune complex-mediated disorders, but it will only be temporary.

The natural way to health recovery?

The attention of scientists in various countries has been directed more and more toward the biochemical method of systemic enzyme therapy. Proponents stress that systemic enzymes are able to cleave and remove pathogenic immune complexes, to stimulate the body's endogenous defenses and to accelerate the mechanisms of inflammation and thereby bring them to an earlier end.

Physicians using enzyme therapy point out, however, that an initial but momentary aggravation of the condition can occur. They postulate that the enzyme mixtures are able to break the immune complexes deposited in the tissues down into smaller sized molecules, and thus lead them back into the bloodstream. The increased presence of immune complexes in the bloodstream can make itself felt in the form of an initial increase in the severity of the disease symptoms. However, they feel that the enzymes, if introduced into the body in the required quantities, can soon cope with the numerous, degraded immune complexes which have been channeled into the bloodstream.

This effect has been subjected to closer study by Professor Steffen from the Institute for Immunology of the University of Vienna. Rabbits with pathogenic immune complexes were treated with a concentrated anti-inflammatory enzyme solution containing the best combination found to be particularly applicable for inflammatory diseases. According to Professor Steffen, the more concentrated the anti-inflammatory enzyme mixtures were, the more the immune complexes were destroyed (Figure 28). Reportedly, all of these complexes had been broken down within hours and the rabbits soon regained their health.

It was also observed by the scientists that the rate of degradation was reduced when the immune complexes contained particularly large quantities of antibodies. This was not a result of a reduced activity of the enzymes, but rather due to the enzyme's action on the antibodies.

The scientists reported that if large quantities of antibody were present in the immune complexes, large quantities were degraded, and the final result was a paradoxical increase in the numbers of immune complexes. However, further studies demonstrated that they were all small immune complexes which were gradually degraded completely as time passed.

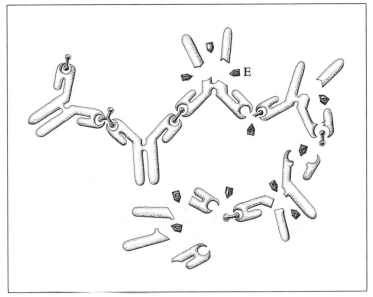

Figure 28: Enzymes cleave an immune complex

All this may seem important for physicians, biochemists and scientifically inclined readers, but the ordinary reader would certainly rather learn which immune complex-mediated diseases can be best treated in this apparently simple manner. It would take too long to list and describe all the diseases treated in Europe and other countries with these methods at present. Let us therefore select just two of the most important autoimmune diseases suitable for this possible aid. We will consider *multiple sclerosis,* which is felt, in part, to be caused by the deposition of immune complexes in the nervous tissue, and *rheumatoid arthritis (chronic polyarthritis)* which is primarily brought about by the deposition of immune complexes in the internal capsule of the joint.

Chapter 10

Multiple sclerosis: The turning point

There are 250,000 known MS patients in the United States (500,000 estimated) according to the National Multiple Sclerosis Society (Rosner and Ross).

The victims of multiple sclerosis must live with the knowledge of the continual worsening of their condition. Anyone who ventures to offer them hope and to say that there is a good chance of diminishing the deterioration or even the effects of the paralysis should be very sure of the facts.

To offer such victims, for whom hopelessness is a constant companion, the possibility of unhoped-for improvement demands a high degree of consciousness of the responsibilities involved. Another disappointment could be a catastrophe for the patient.

European physicians experienced in the use of systemic enzymes strongly believe that, contrary to the usual opinion of physicians utilizing more traditional treatments, a specific group of MS sufferers with active disease whose symptoms get worse by degrees can be helped considerably by treatment based mainly on enzyme therapy.

Now, according to these scientists, it should be considered that there are many experienced physicians worldwide who have been using this systemic enzyme therapy for years, many in controlled studies, and that they are completely and honestly convinced that the extreme suffering of the MS patients can be alleviated with this treatment Based on their research and experience, the physicians in the various studies feel that the progression of the patient's paralysis can be halted, and that many of the symptoms can be alleviated or even disappear.

We are all highly concerned about the health of those who are ill and at the same time feel a deep sense of responsibility to the patients, and to medicine and science. In this regard, the European scientists raise several philosophical questions. They ponder "if we are convinced that a specific and very safe treatment helps, but at the moment do not have all of the scientific proof, how are we to come to terms with denying it to the patients? When we know that we can help them, are we to continue the status quo and wait until we have all of the proof, for the sake of science? Are we thus to allow hundreds of thousands of people throughout the world to continue a life of suffering and a pitiful fate, simply to avoid raising false hopes?"

These scientists are often accused of raising false hopes, and in addition, other arguments used against enzyme therapy for decades are repeated continually, "It cannot possibly work, otherwise everyone would prescribe it." Or the argument, "We don't know the precise cause of multiple sclerosis, so how can these causes be treated? We can therefore do nothing else but tinker with the symptoms in some way, alleviate the pain a little, strengthen the body slightly, and otherwise improve the morale of the patient. Everything else that has been tried, and there have been dozens of enthusiastically accepted approaches to healing MS, has later been found to be somewhat useless." Is this the answer? Well, in reality there are no easy answers. We must all do what in our best judgment and in good conscience is best for the patient, within the limits allowed by law and the government agencies limit what we can do, even if a treatment has been found to be beneficial in other countries.

The search for the error

At present, science has considerable knowledge regarding the mechanisms that may lead us to learn the actual cause of multiple sclerosis. It has naturally been known for a long time that MS victims gradually suffer a functional loss of the central nervous system. This is a result of the demyelination of the nerves. The nerves are surrounded by a layer containing myelin which plays a role in the transmission of the impulse from one nerve to another. In other words, myelin is active in the transfer of messages because it insulates the nerve axons so that the messages can properly bridge the tiny gaps between the nerves. If myelin is lacking, these messages do not reach their destination. The organs affected by this disturbance in nervous conduction can no longer react and are functionally lamed.

There is as yet no agreement as to exactly what causes the myelin of the nerves to cease functioning or to disappear. What is it that brings about inflammation and in the end destroys the nerve sheath? Why does this destruction extend without any recognizable pattern, destroying the function of an organ in one area and then that of another organ?

An inherited predisposition, or genetic susceptibility, may play a role here, but that does not explain what might be genetically altered. At least there is room for discussion here. It has further been suggested that an incorrect diet, lacking in selenium for instance, might lead to this illness. Selenium is a nonmetal that is absolutely essential in trace amounts for some metabolic processes and which the organism cannot produce for itself. We ingest it with our food, but we also breathe it in from the air and take it in through our skin, it is excreted with the urine and stool, and is also expelled with perspiration and through breathing. Selenium is a remarkable hybrid, sometimes acting as an enzyme activator, sometimes as an enzyme inhibitor. However, there is no proof that this is the cause.

It has also been suggested that the ratio of saturated to unsaturated fatty acids in the diet might play a role in the demyelination of the central nerves and there has been a discussion of the consequences which might develop from a disturbed uptake of unsaturated fatty acids.

Finally, it is thought by some that viruses are involved in the destruction of the myelin. Scientists have considered a second attack or reactivation of viruses which have lain dormant in the organism for years after an infection with measles, or perhaps one of the slow virus diseases which can develop into an illness months or even years after infection. Of interest is the fact that MS has been linked to the geographic location where the patient spent the first 15 years of life, where individuals from cold or temperate climates demonstrated a higher incidence than those from the tropics. Genetic factors may influence susceptibility. Relocation after the age 15 does not alter the risk.

During this search for an explanation, it became clear that most MS patients have an unusually high level of immune complexes. This has been confirmed by studies carried out independently in America, Greece, Czechoslovakia and Germany. The serum of MS patients almost always contains considerably higher concentrations of circulating immune complexes than does that of healthy individuals.

This led to the suspicion that MS could be a disease dependent on or even caused by immune complexes, also known as an autoimmune disease (Figure 29). Perhaps all the previously postulated influences, genetic predisposition, selenium deficiency, fatty acid imbalance, viruses, alone or together, lead to a 'mistake within the immune system', to an uncontrolled reaction against the body itself.

Should the body's own unchanged myelin come to be seen as an antigen as a result of such influences, will our antibodies begin to attach themselves to it and will the accumulation of stable immune complexes lead to an attack by the alarmed complement cascade resulting further in damage to the neighboring nerve tissue and to the myelin? The results of research published by several institutes tend to support this theory. A medical team at the Neurological Institute of Würzburg University, in Germany, for example, has actually detected antibodies that are directed against myelin, and attach themselves to it to form immune complexes.

It is still too soon to maintain that we know for certain what causes multiple sclerosis, but we can state with a clear conscience that immune complexes of a particular size and type, and in certain concentrations, play a role in the disease and appear to be associated with the increased severity of the disease. It also has

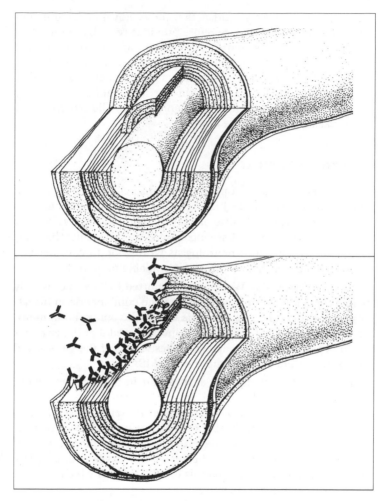

Figure 29: Development of multiple sclerosis
     Above: Healthy nerve surrounded by a multilayered myelin sheath
     Below: Antibodies have become attached to the myelin and destruction
                  begins

been suggested by the scientists that the removal of these pathogenic immune complexes therefore provides relief by interrupting the progressive deterioration and even, among other things, reversing the loss of function of individual nerves. An interesting theory? The theory has considerable support in clinical practice. This is observed, for example, in the plasmapheresis already described, where the immune complexes are filtered from the blood plasma outside of the body.

The best verification?

German and other European physicians believe that the role of immune complexes in MS has been demonstrated for almost two decades now through the use of enzyme therapy. The results were very impressive. They feel so encouraged by the results that they have made an appeal to neurologists worldwide to consider this therapeutic approach and to make it available to more patients.

Even Professor Max Wolf himself reported to have successfully treated some MS patients with his enzyme combination in his latter years. At that time, however, he was of the opinion that multiple sclerosis was caused by viruses and assumed that the enzymes would degrade the proteinaceous adhesiveness of the viruses and thereby inactivate them to improve the MS.

It is unlikely that there is a physician in practice with more experience in the field of MS treatment than Dr. Neuhofer in Salzburg, Austria, who as an MS sufferer herself has been able to limit the progress of the disease with the most potent enzyme mixture. She or her colleagues have thus far treated more than 350 MS patients according to a scheme she has developed. In 1986, she published a statistical analysis of 150 patients which she had treated with hydrolytic enzymes.

Her patients were generally recommended to follow a special diet with a high proportion of raw foodstuffs and only polyunsaturated fatty acids.

Otherwise, they usually only received a potent oral enzyme mixture. Specific criteria were employed to decide on the dosage of the enzymes, which specific preparation, in what form and at what point in time it should be administered to the patient. During acute stages, the oral enzymes were supplemented with injectable enzymes.

Made-to-order MS treatment

Multiple sclerosis is a disease that expresses itself quite individually. There is virtually no uniform disease pattern. Every MS patient exhibits a 'personal MS' which differs somewhat or even considerably in its manifestation and course from the MS of all other sufferers. Therefore, according to Dr. Neuhofer, the whole art of treating MS with enzymes depends on taking account of this individuality, on taking the right steps at exactly the right time and with the right dosage.

It depends on whether the disease progresses intermittently, in other words, whether there are intervals of at least four weeks between acute phases, or whether an initially intermittent progression converts to a chronic, uniformly developing disorder. It also depends on which nerves have already failed, how rapidly the disease is progressing, how long it has been present and many other factors.

In addition, the question of how long and with which medications a particular patient has been treated previously is decisive for the choice of, and for the success of the treatment. For example, to what state the immune surveillance of the patient has been compromised by using drugs that weaken the immune system, for instance such immunosuppressives as the well-known, cortisone-containing drugs or anticancer agents?

The results of Dr. Neuhofer's first 150 patient treatments which she has analyzed allow some conclusions concerning which cases can be expected to yield favorable results and which are accompanied by a less favorable prognosis.

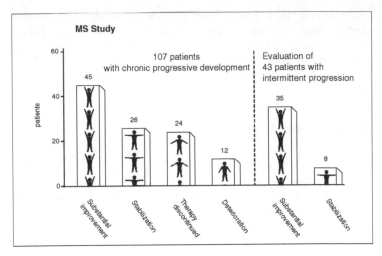

Figure 30: Results of the Neuhofer study on enzyme treatment in MS patients

From a total of 107 patients suffering from chronic progressive multiple sclerosis, 24 patients broke off treatment because their health insurance would not bear the costs. From a total of 83 patients who were fully evaluated, 71 improved, with 45 cases demonstrating a substantial improvement, and 26 patients revealed a slowing in the progression of the illness. The patient's condition deteriorated in only 12 cases, all of whom had previously received long-term treatment with a substance which suppresses the body's own immune system (azathioprine).

Dr. Neuhofer's results are quite impressive, and should be carefully evaluated and confirmed by repeated studies. Her results are particularly encouraging since they were as good or better than any other statistical findings in this field (Figure 30).

What is the effect of the orally administered or intramuscularly injected enzyme mixtures on *intermittent, progressive MS*? Can the enzymes exert any inhibitory effect at all when the progression in deterioration is also accompanied by an intermittent increase in the level of immune complexes?

The results were surprising. Dr. Neuhofer's statistics reveal that of the 43 patients suffering from this intermittent progression, almost all, namely 35, demonstrated substantial improvement, with some cases going as far as the reversal of all symptoms of paralysis. The conditions of the remaining 8 patients were at least stabilized (Figure 30).

In the intermittently progressive group, not one single patient was observed who suffered a deterioration of symptoms during therapy. There were no serious side effects found. Some patients developed occasional local reddening and swelling at the site of enzyme injection.

Other physicians have since adopted the scheme worked out by Dr. Neuhofer. Many report similar positive results. Rarely, patients did not respond. Closer investigation of the disappointing cases by the scientists revealed that the treatment schemes required for the particular case had not been carried out accurately. For instance, according to Dr. Neuhofer, it is essential that immediate intramuscular enzyme injections take place at the first signs of a new phase in cases where the MS progresses intermittently. If this is neglected for even one or two days, it is impossible to affect the deteriorative phase.

It is not always the physician who is at fault; a patient who is scared of injections or procedures will often delay visiting the physician because the prospect of an intramuscular injection of the enzyme mixtures is not very pleasant.

Dr. Neuhofer and other neurologists experienced in the medical treatment of MS with enzymes explain that there are perhaps three reasons why the enzyme therapy is not generally used for multiple sclerosis: The first is its rejection by established medical practitioners who are reluctant to deviate from conventional teaching and shirk from objectively considering and testing a new treatment scheme on a broader basis, even in the obvious absence of superior alternatives. Secondly, there is the necessity of adapting to the individual realities of each case that excludes a standard prescription of 'a specific number of tablets three times a day', and thus demands a great deal of flexibility, patience and understanding of the individual patient, and of the immune processes coming into play. The third reason is that the patient himself/herself is not always prepared to carry out a precise, consistent, exact therapy and to cooperate, thereby ensuring that this therapy is carried out consistently and optimally.

On account of all this, we are a long way from being able to speak of a complete victory over multiple sclerosis. However, what we can and indeed must speak about to patients is to get motivated in order to achieve a victory over the inactive hopelessness.

Chapter 11

Arthritis and related disorders:
Rheumatic joints: Patience rewarded

It would almost be possible to end the discussion of the enzyme therapy of rheumatic joints here and now, simply by saying, 'See multiple sclerosis'. The similarities between rheumatism and multiple sclerosis are genuinely amazing.

Rheumatism or arthritis refers to a group of conditions affecting primarily the joints, muscles, tendons and soft tissues. Arthritis is a common disorder of variable severity, often associated with severe discomfort, pain and, in some cases, progressive disability. In the United States, it has been estimated that 37,000,000 Americans are affected with some form of arthritis, from very mild to severe. This represents one in seven persons. Two million of these are felt to have rheumatoid arthritis. It is more common in women. Osteoarthritis affects 16 million people. Considering its impact on absenteeism, lost wages and medical care expenses, arthritis costs 35 billion dollars per year in the United States alone.

Thus, rheumatism of the joints includes chronic degenerative joint disease (osteoarthritis) as the 'wear and tear' that comes with aging. It also includes a more severe and disabling disease also referred to as rheumatoid arthritis (Figure 31) or chronic polyarthritis. Rheumatoid arthritis is a disease whose exact cause is also unknown. Hundreds of scientific publications confirm that it is also a disease associated with elevated levels of immune complexes circulating in the blood. It is a disease which is generally treated with immunosuppressive or anti-inflammatory agents. It is a disease where these methods bring about only rather unsatisfactory levels of success and where they are also associated with high risks of side effects. Finally, the European physicians are convinced that it is a disease which can improve, or at least be delayed in its development by means of high-dose or long-term enzyme administration.

Of course, there are some differences from multiple sclerosis which make it worthwhile to go into the matter more deeply. The most important difference is naturally the mental trauma which the MS patient is subjected to. This may be no consolation to the rheumatic patient waking up each morning with stiff painful finger joints and seeing these joints become more and more deformed until the fingers can scarcely be used anymore. But, nevertheless, the prognosis is better than for MS patients and the patient can live to an older age with this disease. In rheumatoid arthritis, although a significant and often disabling problem, the loss of mobility and pain in rheumatoid arthritis are not as devastating as the dramatic loss of one vital function after another that the MS patient is confronted with.

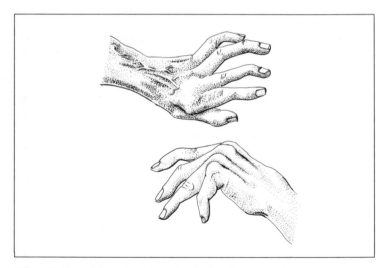

Figure 31: Typical finger joint alterations in chronic articular rheumatism

Another difference is that there are many more patients with rheumatism than there are sufferers from MS and the treatment of rheumatic joints therefore affects more people. For this reason, there are more scientific studies and publications, and considerably more practical experiences with treatment.

Naturally, there are also certain differences in the mechanisms leading to the immune complex-mediated destruction of the myelin in the nervous system, and by which the immune complexes entering the internal capsule of the joint bring about the destruction of the finger and toe joints (Figure 31).

Let us spare ourselves a description of this phenomenon which would only lead us deeper and deeper into the difficult field of immunology. Let us be satisfied with the knowledge that rheumatoid arthritis is associated again and again with increases in the level of immune complexes. Nowadays, this can be measured very well.

Last, but not least, it is possible to establish the degree of rheumatic risk, or of developing rheumatic disease, from the immune complexes measured with the help of the rheumatoid factor. Let us quote freely from the work of one of the authors (Miehlke), a rheumatologist, "Immune complexes themselves act as antigens and provoke the plasma cells to synthesize antibodies against the gamma globulins contained in these immune complexes." The so-formed autoantibodies are also referred to as rheumatoid factors.

The rheumatoid factor with which all physicians are familiar, even those who do not personally concern themselves with this complicated ping pong game between antigen, antibody and autoantibody, has lead many physicians to consider very carefully the thoughts of enzymologists who maintain that rheumatism is associated with the formation of pathogenic immune complexes. These enzymologists also maintain that the disease could be considerably alleviated by the detection, degradation and disposal of the immune complexes which have penetrated the joint cartilage by way of the synovial fluid.

This should actually be of interest to every physician. Patients suffering from rheumatism form the bread and butter of many physicians, particularly general practitioners, with patients visiting the practice dutifully for years, since rheumatism is probably one of the most chronic of all chronic diseases.

Unfortunately, there is not a very broad choice of effective therapeutic measures. It has become even more reduced in recent years since the long-term administration of cortisone-containing preparations and other anti-inflammatory substances has had to be severely curtailed. Steroid hormones actually alleviate the patients' symptoms relatively quickly and can also stop the progression of joint deterioration. However, this results via a suppression of the body's own defenses which can in the long run lead to disorders which are more serious than the rheumatism which is being treated.

Nonsteroidal anti-inflammatories, such as ibuprofen, are also able to alleviate the pain and other symptoms of inflammation, but they have no effect on the progressive degeneration of the joint. Their action depends on the inhibition of the substance prostaglandin which plays a mediatory role in the development of inflammations. However, since nature does not just produce a black-and-white picture, this prostaglandin plays both a positive as well as a negative role in the processes within our bodies. Thus, it protects the mucosa of the gastrointestinal tract from attack by the stomach acids, meaning that prostaglandin-inhibiting drugs can cause inflammation, bleeding and ulcers of the gastrointestinal tract. In addition, these drugs can cause depletion of platelets, the essential clotting elements, and this can also lead to gastrointestinal bleeding.

Many suffer and few are helped

In addition to the immunosuppressant drugs, the physician can make use of what are called basic anti-rheumatic therapeutic preparations. There is a small group of such substances that reduces the number of immune complexes and neutralizes their effects by mechanisms which are not always clear. They are injected intramuscularly, administered orally or injected directly into the affected joint.

The best-known basic therapeutic agent is probably *gold*. Gold has been used as a drug since antiquity to treat tuberculosis, leprosy and syphilis, among other things. Afterall, alchemists tried to transmute gold into potable gold, a heal-all substance which is the subject in thousands of myths. It was not known how it functioned as a remedy, but everyone was convinced that it did.

In rheumatology today, gold is administered to the patient in the form of organogold compounds. We still do not know how gold works, but it is still prescribed. Unfortunately, every third patient receiving intramuscular gold injections suffers side effects, and these can be very substantial. In addition, medical reports indicate that long-term administration of gold accumulates in the tissues, can act as a vascular toxin, can cause allergic skin changes and lead to illnesses of the eye, anemia and a series of other side effects.

Penicillamine is frequently administered to counteract the side effects of gold. However, penicillamine is itself a basic therapeutic agent in its own right and is therefore subject to risks similar to those associated with gold. Thus, all that happens is that the cause of side effects are exchanged.

Once, during a continuing medical education conference, Dr. Brückle, rheumatology professor of the University of Basel, reported to his not particularly enthused colleagues what the basic antirheumatic therapy prescribed day by day in medical practices throughout the world means to the patient. According to him, the reported success rates of up to 40% simply did not stand up to further examination. Medical reports revealed that the actual figures are much lower. Only in one of every six patients whose symptoms are improved does this improvement persist for more than two years. More precisely, it is calculated today that the improvement rate is about 19% for gold and 17% for penicillamine. This improvement lasts an average of about ten months. The longer the patient has been suffering rheumatic symptoms, the smaller the chance that such drugs will have any effect at all, and they may instead precipitate side effects, some of which may be dangerous.

Should the joint degeneration continue in spite of these therapeutics, the next stage is the prescription of cytostatics which inhibit cell production and therefore also the production of antibodies. In this way, they are able to inhibit the production of new immune complexes while at the same time, unfortunately, they stop the production of new cells for the continual renewal of the body.

The most frequently prescribed of these drugs is azathioprine. It has already been described by Dr. Neuhofer how powerfully it hinders the attempted enzymatic treatment of immune complex diseases in the case of multiple sclerosis. The serious side effects of azathioprine, where particularly the formation of blood cells can be disrupted, often force the therapy to be abandoned.

It is no wonder that many patients refuse to take such drugs. Thus, according to Dr. Brückle, about three quarters of all patients with rheumatoid arthritis abandon basic therapy on their own accord within two years.

Physicians who are seriously interested in a more effective, less harmful remedy for their unfortunate rheumatic patients are undoubtedly disheartened as well. It is only too understandable that the specialist world is filled with the cry, "At last we have it! The drug that gets right to the cause of rheumatism has been found!"

With this goal, investigators have even dug out century old herbal remedies from volumes in monastery libraries. There is enthusiasm when something like omega-3-fatty acid turns up; some fish are particularly rich in it and it has an effect under certain circumstances. Afterall, the fatty acid is polyunsaturated and such a deficiency may be a contributing factor in the production of pathogenic immune complexes, as has already been discussed in the case of multiple sclerosis.

Whether the enzyme mixtures are the drug longed-for to get at the cause of such rheumatic diseases as rheumatoid arthritis is also the subject of discussion. What is certain, however, is that, in the experience of one of the authors (Miehlke), enzyme preparations are as good as, or superior to, other anti-rheumatic agents on account of their comparable efficacy and their lack of dangerous side effects.

Physicians who are searching so desperately for an alternative to today's treatments should pay special attention to the studies and reports of systemic enzymes for rheumatologic conditions. They appear as a viable therapeutic possibility. Perhaps, when they read the reports detailing how remarkable these enzymes appear to be in destroying the pathogenic immune complexes, they simply will find it difficult to believe. Or perhaps, despite the low effectiveness of the traditional treatments, they are afraid of litigation if they step outside the traditional dogma. We hope that this book will motivate them to investigate this treatment. If they find it is not effective, that in itself will be a contribution. Afterall, rheumatology has not been truly blessed with good therapeutic news.

More precious than gold

One of the pieces of good news will therefore be repeated here. In a clinical study lasting six months, the head professor of the Rehabilitation Center for Rheumatic Disorders and Cardiovascular Disease in Saalfelden, Austria, Dr. Klein, reported their studies demonstrating that the effect of taking such combinations as the anti-inflammatory enzyme mixtures was just as great as the effect of gold. At present, gold is regarded as probably the best and safest basic therapy available for rheumatoid arthritis sufferers. In contrast to the gold group, the group receiving the anti-inflammatory enzyme mixtures included more rheumatic patients in advanced stages who had been suffering from the disease for a longer period. It is known that the chances of healing the disorder decrease with each additional year's duration of the illness. Thus, the reported responses in advanced stages and long duration disease already represent successes for the anti-inflammatory enzyme mixtures.

However, what impressed Professor Klein even more during this study was that the anti-inflammatory enzyme mixtures demonstrated an appreciably improved tolerance. While 20% of the patients treated with gold complained of side effects, only 5% of the patients treated with the anti-inflammatory enzyme mixtures were dissatisfied, and this was primarily because of the number of tablets required, loose bowel and the smell of the stool. According to Professor Klein, the difference in side effects, in itself, ought to provide sufficient reason for considering the anti-inflammatory enzyme mixtures, which their studies showed to be equal in efficacy, but superior with respect to tolerance.

The scientific publications collected by the Medical Enzyme Research Institute, as well as current scientific investigations, report that, "enzyme preparations such as the original Wolf anti-inflammatory mixture, or the related rheumatologic enzyme preparation, are not only virtually free from side effects, but that their clinical effects are as favorable or better than those of oral gold or other basic therapeutic preparations."

They indicate that the enzymes can be used to alleviate the symptoms in rheumatologic disorders, including such external signs as morning stiffness, pain, joint swelling, loss of grip strength and the ability to bend the joints.

They also claim that enzymes affect an additional and specific mechanism, whose importance is often not properly recognized, and which is at least indirectly associated with the cause of rheumatic disease. This refers to a fibrin mantle which develops around immune complexes as a natural attempt of the body to isolate the problem area, but which unfortunately serves to prevent the complexes from being reached by the other body defenses. The researchers report that the enzymes degrade the fibrin mantle built up around the tissue-bound immune complexes, and thus remove their cloak of invisibility. Thereafter, enzymes allow the immune complexes to be actively degraded by the natural body defenses. With the help of the enzymes themselves, they are then broken down and separated from the tissue matrix, and thereby eliminated. The researchers postulate that, in this manner, the mechanisms leading to inflammation are cut off more rapidly and further tissue deterioration is halted.

Over the years, the results of a series of clinical investigations have been published confirming that enzyme compounds are actually capable of removing circulating immune complexes from the blood serum of rheumatic patients. These investigations also report that favorable clinical results accompany these changes.

Thus, in 1983, a clinical report was published presenting the results of a large-scale study involving the treatment of 1,004 rheumatic patients with the rheumatologic enzyme mixture. The group covered patients with rheumatic joint disease of various types, including cases of rheumatoid arthritis as well as soft tissue rheumatism , osteoarthritis and many other types of rheumatic disability. Afterall, the term rheumatism covers dozens of quite different disorders of the musculoskeletal system, from muscle inflammation to ordinary arthritis and up to and including deforming arthritis of the spine, namely ankylosing spondylitis.

In various published reports of multicenter, methodical and carefully conducted studies, the rheumatologic enzyme mixtures were used by 141 physicians to treat 1,004 patients. The case histories were documented and evaluated. The results were impressive. Depending on the particular rheumatic disorder, the therapists classified 76 to 96% of patients as improved or considerably improved. The condition remained unchanged in 10 to 24% of patients and only 2% suffered a deterioration of their condition. The opinion of the patients concerning the success of treatment was almost identical. The overwhelming majority of patients and physicians evaluated the rheumatologic enzyme mixtures as being 'excellent' or 'good'. The proportion of patients who tolerated the enzyme mixtures poorly was less than 1%.

Reports from studies in Austria by the Institute for Immunology in Vienna, and in Germany by the Rheumatology Clinic in Wiesbaden, and the Rheumatology Clinic in Bad Wiessee, have also reached similar conclusions. They have indicated that it is possible to successfully treat various forms of rheumatism with enzymes. The authors claimed that the enzymes partially, but significantly, reduced limitations in movement and alleviated pain. They reported that it is at least possible to slow down or completely halt the continually progressing deterioration of the joints and related tissues. The postulated mechanism of action was via a direct action on the immune system.

A happy outcome

All this sounds virtually unbelievable! A method of treatment that brings such remarkable results and is so free from side effects must have some disadvantage or another.

There have been several publications by the Medical Enzymes Research Institute also concerned with the possible disadvantages of enzyme therapy. According to their reports, the most remarkable disadvantage of the rheumatologic enzyme mixtures is their delayed effect. They point out that one must expect the treatment of a disorder which has been developing for many years will not yield dramatic changes within a short period of time measured in weeks, and patients must not be bitterly disappointed if health is not restored immediately. They reported that it could be that the patient has to take the rheumatologic enzyme mixtures for weeks or even months before a positive effect appears. According to them, this means that the patient must continue to bear the pain and accept the limitations in mobility day in, day out, but must continue to take the rheumatologic enzyme mixture tablets, initially without any disheartening response. And not just a few of them, the required dose being from 6 to 30 tablets per day, depending on the mixture taken. Some patients reject this on account of the fact that they have been warned time and again not to take too many 'chemical' substances. However, the enzyme scientists further state that, "the whole point in this case is that there are no 'chemical' substances here, but that they are such natural, biological aids as those produced by the body itself."

At present, in the United States, enzyme treatment for rheumatic diseases is not an available option. In countries where enzyme treatment is available, rheumatism therefore demands great patience by the patient initially. Also perseverance. And money, since some health insurance policies still refuse to cover a share in the cost of this treatment.

Health insurance will pay for even more expensive medications as long as they are not considered experimental, or are 'approved' by the FDA in the U.S. or the equivalent agencies in other countries. If and once enzyme treatments are fully accepted by the traditional medicine for what they are, another reasonable and valid therapeutic option it is to be expected, that it will be covered by insurance plans. In addition, when a drug works and helps for certain diseases, perseverance on the part of the patient might eventually lead to political changes, and subsequently to proper research and the eventual approval of a drug. In Europe, should the patient have to bear the costs personally, they amount to approximately the daily cost of cigarettes for a smoker.

Another aspect of the treatment regarded by some as a disadvantage is the absolute requirement for dose adjustments depending on the activity of the disease. This demands alert attentiveness by both the patient and physician concerning the status of the illness, and adjustment of the dosages in a timely manner when required, if success is truly sought, as is customary with systemic steroids. Just as with multiple sclerosis, it is absolutely essential when treating inflammatory rheumatism that the patient go straight to the physician the day it becomes evident a new episode of activity is beginning; when the patient feels a cold, a flu or some other infection coming on (which in many patients trigger flares) or otherwise does not feel well. Under such circumstances, the maintenance dose of the rheumatologic enzyme mixture tablets is no longer sufficient since higher doses of enzymes are required. Thus, there are physicians who report excellent results if they increase the dosage, particularly if they inject proper dosages of the more potent enzyme mixtures intramuscularly at the first signs of a new phase of rheumatic activity. Some patients dread this because they do not like the injections. The continuation and further deterioration of the rheumatic condition, however, is even more unpleasant.

Enzymologists believe the reason the greatly increased dose is important is that larger numbers of immune complexes are to be found in the synovial fluid, in the cartilage of the affected joint and in the blood at this time. If the body is given a sufficient dose of enzymes, they can attack the immune complexes and thus carry out a sort of spring cleaning exercise. It also promotes the 'good inflammation'. Why? Doesn't inflammation lead to joint damage? This is both correct and incorrect at one and the same time. Inflammation is rather different than it is normally thought to be. The proper degree of inflammation is actually beneficial. It is just that it has to be held within certain limits, beyond which it should be brought to an end more quickly. The enzymes ensure this, they believe. They claim that this is one of the decisive advantages of enzyme therapy.

Chapter 12

Inflammation: A beneficial process
Healing, cleaning and repair

It is quite simple. Everyone is well aware what an inflammation is; if a wound gets hot, turns red, hurts and swells, that is an inflammation. But most people do not know that there are subliminal or 'good inflammations' constantly occurring in our bodies which protect us and help repair any damage.

To most people 'inflammations' are those unpleasant, usually painful disorders ranging from appendicitis to nephritis, from a tonsillitis to a pyelonephritis; every medical speciality encounters them. We are all aware of them, but do we understand them?

On the contrary! We do not understand them as well as we think when we attempt to describe what is taking place in the body while inflammation occurs. Otherwise we would all know that inflammation is not a disease, but rather just the opposite, it is a sign that healing and repair are occurring, through at least three beneficial processes which are absolutely essential for recovery. The *first* is the fight against the pathogen or offender, the *second*, after the battle, is to clear the damaged area from the resulting impurities and toxins, and the *third* is the repair and reconstitution of the damaged site. The mechanism by which all this is performed is so amazing, so ingenious that we have to admire the capabilities of our bodies. Let us follow such a process in outline and, for clarity, we will leave out some of the details which could possibly lead to controversy and criticism.

Alarm at every wound

Let us take an example. Imagine that you got a splinter in your finger and could not remove every last piece; a tiny fragment remains in the wound. The region then becomes inflamed. The process always follows the same pattern if the body is exposed to a damaging influence. A nerve stimulus is first transmitted and alarms the organism stimulating a fantastic, combined defense operation by a multitude of various systems.

There are a multitude of similar but more damaging influences which lead to inflammation. Just to list a few, these include wounds, heat (burns), physical irritation (friction, chronic sores) or radiation (e.g., X-rays, cobalt irradiation, even sunburn or chronic ultraviolet light damage). Also chemical irritation, poisons, gases, and foreign bodies. It could be a microbiological invasion by viruses, bacteria, parasites or fungi as well, or a substance precipitating an allergy, or the immune complexes we have already discussed. Or it could be a cell turning cancerous. Unfortunately, the list is almost endless.

Whatever causes the damage, it first alerts the troops that undertake our surveillance and protection to limit the damage and then to destroy what is causing the damage, to clear up the damaged area, to clean and finally to repair everything, and ultimately to restore a good state of health. We recognize the perceptible and the occasionally visible signs of this rescue service, the redness, swelling, heat and pain, as the signs of inflammation, and usually mistake them for the disorder.

Rescue is not yet at hand in the example we have chosen, since a tiny splinter is still in the finger. The splinter caused the affected nerves to relay a pain stimulus and this can actually be measured in the form of a sort of shock reaction of the blood vessels. The blood vessels in the region of the lesion first contract for half a second or perhaps half a minute, depending on the stimulus. And then it begins. Your body has noticed that something has happened and where the damage has taken place. It now requires specific white blood cells, the famous leukocytes of the cellular defenses, to advance against the foreign matter at the site of the wound. Furthermore, it requires many macrophages to devour the intruder and for cleaning up the lesion. Thrombocytes are also necessary to make the blood in the wound clot, thereby limiting the damage to this region.

All these helpers are constantly swimming in the pool of blood and lymph so that even as the smallest vessel is damaged by the splinter, they emerge from that vessel and make themselves useful. These few are naturally not enough. The organism requires enormous numbers for repair and regeneration. Depending on the cause, the repair may be accomplished quickly or may take a long time to finish the job.

Get the little devils going

The technical problem that the body has to solve first, therefore, is how to get as many as possible of the lymphocytes, macrophages and thrombocytes, and a half dozen other helpers circulating in the blood and lymph, transported as rapidly as possible out of the vessels and into the region of the lesion. How can the helpers already in the region of the lesion be stimulated to the highest state of activity?

The organism carries this out in a very clever manner. It activates messengers in the smallest blood vessels around the lesion, which in turn are able to dilate these vessels. These capillaries are extremely fine and supply each and every cell with energy-giving, oxygen-saturated blood. This is referred to as the microcirculation. 'Dilation' is perhaps the wrong word since these little blood vessels are not puffed up, which in itself would hardly be possible. What happens is that the individual cells of the capillaries which are normally packed closely together are caused to move somewhat apart by the messengers so that the microcirculation system becomes as porous as a sponge.

In any case, the primary reaction normally takes place during the first four hours after damage occurs. The blood vessels in the tissue surrounding the damaged or destroyed area become more permeable, the helpers called up to destroy or remove the enemy, to seal off the damaged region, to break up the debris and to clear up the battlefield, can get to their work. They swim around together in the region of the lesion in a blood tinged fluid which also flows through the interstices that have appeared between the cells of the blood vessels.

Everyone is familiar with this colorless fluid, it is sometimes formed when a wound 'oozes'. Sometimes, it can happen that the wound contains damaging enemies from the environment, bacteria for instance, which thrive on this exudate and carry on with their damaging activity. The initial fluid then becomes an exudate which has been enriched with clotting factors, cell debris, dead and living enemies. The body expels it whenever there is an opportunity. We call this exudate pus.

Everyone who has ploughed so far through this book will have realized that none of the work of degradation and sealing-off carried out by the cells could take place without enzymes. Many cascades of enzyme reactions are activated one after another. These include the enzyme cascade of complement, leading to the final, primed, ninth component of this complement, the deadly killer.

The four classical signs

The region swells more and more, since ever more fluid accompanies the helping cells through the deliberate leaks in the capillary blood vessels surrounding the wound. You can see this in the case of your finger, the site where the splinter is still embedded. It swells over the first few hours. In any type of inflammation, this swelling varies in extent depending on the site, nature and severity of the injury.

Reddening also appears. This reddening is naturally a result of the increased blood flow to the site of the injury which leads to an overheating of the area as well.

In the case of a particularly fierce battle between the forces that have been summoned and the locally fixed intruder (Figure 32), a localized heat reaction develops, precipitated by the various defense messengers already discussed. If all their efforts cannot

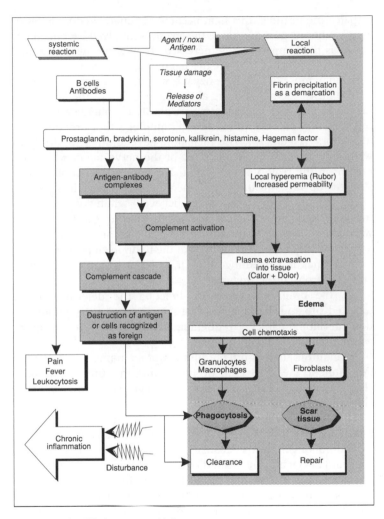

Figure 32: Simplified sequence of inflammatory events

displace the intruder, this heat becomes a generalized body fever. This too has its purpose, since the enzmyes involved become more active as the temperature is increased. They work away like mad at about 40 °C (104 °F), but the temperature cannot increase by very much more or else the enzymes will 'die'.

The messengers that bring about the opening of the intracellular spaces and cause overheating are absolutely mandatory for the inflammatory process. In medical terminology, they are known as 'mediators' (Figure 32). The mediators have another job to do as well, they alert the pain receptors of the nerve fibers which are present in the region of the lesion. The nerves then conduct this stimulus upwards to the brain's nerve center where it is experienced as pain. Even if you cannot believe it when you are suffering pain, this is an important and helpful mechanism. The brain is warned that there is a situation which is dangerous to health, that an enemy has entered the body, that the brain itself perhaps ought to intervene, do something about it, in order to protect the body and itself from further invasions.

So, the brain intervenes in directing the defenses to the required site and the four classical symptoms of every inflammation develop, namely, reddening (rubor), swelling (tumor), warmth (calor) and pain (dolor).

In addition, there is often a fifth symptom, namely loss of function (functio laesa). It is to be hoped that this fifth symptom is absent as a result of the splinter in your finger, since you can probably still move your finger.

The first emergency measures are completed between the fourth and twelfth hour after the splinter entered your finger. The wound no longer bleeds because the blood flow has been deliberately and enzymatically pushed out of equilibrium in the direction of coagulation. The sealing-off of the lesion from the surrounding healthy tissue is also complete. The necessary helpers have congregated where they are needed to degrade the tissue debris in the region of the wound and then to liquefy it, so that it can be transported away.

Clean-up and renovation

Strictly speaking, the breakdown and removal of tissue debris is an activity directed against the body's own tissue. The enzymes degrade something that is our own protein. They consume a part of us. How can that be possible? When our cells are destroyed as a result of injury or due to an attack by an enemy, they lose the markers that indicate they are part of our own body as they die. They develop their own antigenic properties and thereby change into 'foreign bodies'. It therefore becomes clear to our enzymes that it is quite in order for them to degrade and remove these foreign cells.

Sometimes it takes a few hours before the cells in the region of a wound die off properly and without question become foreign. For this reason, the process of cleaning-up the tissue debris at the site of a lesion does not begin immediately. Naturally, the enzymes can begin from the very first minutes to act against foreign bodies consisting of proteins which have penetrated into the wound, against viruses, bacteria and other microorganisms. They carry out this task in an exemplary manner.

From between 12 and 36 hours after the lesion has occurred, the process of degradation, liquefaction and removal goes on incessantly (Figures 17 and 32). At the same time, almost incidentally, regeneration commences in the sealed-off, cleaned-up area of the wound. This is the result of special neurotransmission or 'electrical impulses' at the tips of the nerve fibers reaching into the wound. These fibers grow a short distance into the wound and primitive cells (alone able to do nothing, yet capable of everything) begin to form as a result of the electrical impulses.

These cells are rather like those developed as human life commences in the mother's womb. Each of these 'pluripotential' cells has the genetic capability of producing new cells which can mature to produce a specific cell line, with a limited function, within the organism. Scientists also believe that these cells can contribute to the formation of a body organ, or theoretically a whole new individual, or an exact copy of each person. In real life, this does not quite happen to this extent because enzyme inhibitors stop the chain of events when the repair or mission has been completed. This transformation of an undifferentiated into a differentiated cell takes place by means of the enzyme-initiated blockage of particular hereditary regions within the cell until only the program actually required for cell specification remains active.

It would be tempting to begin an exciting description of the mechanism of restoration of damaged tissue, devastated organs, or the theoretical possibility of regrowing amputated limbs, but that is a completely different topic. Furthermore, the splinter is still in the wound and must be removed.

Removal normally occurs in the damaged area during the restorative phase. However, it is sometimes not very easy for your body to expel such a mechanical irritant as a splinter. The splinter has to be isolated and then pushed to the surface by a collection of solidified exudate. This requires fantastically complicated processes involving blood coagulation, blood liquefaction, swelling and shrinkage of the area (Figures 31 and 32) It is no wonder that even a tiny splinter can occasionally cause very severe pain. This is not just because the mediators report to the pain receptors, it also depends on the purely mechanical pressure on the nerve ends. However, it is this strong pressure which ensures that the splinter reaches the surface where we sometimes notice it for the first time days after it entered the finger and finally remove it entirely with a needle or tweezers. Otherwise, all that is involved is healing. This means cell regeneration, new nerve fibers, blood and lymph vessels to supply the new tissue cells being formed at the site of the lesion.

The rescue brigades which were called up and which brought about the inflammation have now finished their work. The permeable microcirculation has long since been sealed off, the exudate has been transported from the wound, the swelling has gone down, the reddening has faded, the pain has stopped. The enzymes that dissolve clotted blood have also completed their work long ago. The conditions in the region of the lesion have normalized.

When the restoration of healthy tissue at the site of the wound is complete, the scab protecting the lesion from further external enemies can fall away. The injury is forgotten.

The inflammation caused by a tiny splinter is an example of an acute inflammation which leads to a complete restoration of the original state. Unfortunately, this does not always happen since it is not always possible to bring about complete renewal. Occasionally, if the foreign body cannot be dissolved or expelled within a reasonable period of time, the body surrounds it with specialized cells that allow the gradual breakdown into smaller components and eventual removal over a period of months or years. This slower process we call *granulomatous inflammation.*

Other times, upon resolution of the inflammation and repair of the damaged site, the newly produced cells are of inferior quality or perhaps simply too many cells are produced. The result is nobby scar tissue. If excessive, a *keloid scar* is formed.

Errors, defects, chaos

An acute inflammation sometimes develops into a chronic inflammation. What then occurs is that there are successive processes of alarm, combat, damage, clean-up and regeneration of some disturbance or another. The stimulus triggering the alarm can be too weak or it can be that the troops deployed for battle, clean-up and renovation are not strong enough because the required number of helpers are not available. The organism then tries to make up for this by means of what is known as a secondary inflammatory reaction in which the whole body is affected. The mediators stimulating overheating are set into action to produce a proper fever. The local measures no longer suffice and the whole body is brought to the highest level of activity to supply enzymes.

The composition of the blood is measurably changed as well. It contains ever more lymphocytes, macrophages, thrombocytes and other helpers. These helpers or mediators are necessary to produce a 'good inflammation', and their concentration in the blood is used medically to grade the type and severity of the accompanying immune reaction.

The violence of the attack by the pathogen can naturally be a reason for the body's inadequate response as well. This can be a result of the virulence of the pathogen or the quantity of pathogen involved. Many factors are known that can convert an acute inflammation into a chronic one.

One factor which is certainly always involved in the chronic inflammation, and the reader will no longer be surprised to learn, is a shortage of the required enzymes. All inflammation reactions are absolutely dependent on the presence of such enzymes. When the scale of damage is large, or the pathogen persistent, the internal support enzymes are required in quantities which the body is unable to produce for itself. The body cannot alter its rate of enzyme production greatly, it cannot simply put its foot down on the accelerator or the brake at will.

Should the body's defense system's internal enzyme shortage cause a breakdown in the complicated chain of interlocking reactions involved in removing the damage and restoring the healthy state, the result is chaos. There is no longer a regulated progression, no planned sequence from the first alarm to the formation of the last new cell. Many of the reactions become intermingled, cancel each other out, or hamper one another. The body tissues themselves loose their markers and the body regards them as foreign enemies, setting yet another defense against them, often called *autoimmunity* or *autoaggression*. This means that our own defenses are now fighting our own cells which are no longer recognized as part of the 'self' because they have lost their normal identity markers. This autoimmunity leads to our own body attacking specific tissues, like the joints, the skin, the connective tissue, the blood cells, or other important areas. Meanwhile, the original cause of the inflammation and damage is unaffected, and it can therefore continue to carry on its destructive work.

This also means that a vicious circle of damaging irritation and autoaggression is set up at the incompletely healed lesion and that this situation builds to an ever more dangerous process, leading ultimately to chronic illnesses which may linger indefinitely, or in other cases can only be interrupted or healed with difficulty.

Traditional medicine often employs different medications under these conditions, in order to slow down the body's own defenses. The doctor may try to stop the action of the inflammation inducing mediators using the prostaglandin inhibitors described in the chapter on rheumatic joints. For more severe cases, physicians use cortisone or other immune suppressive medications.

Under these conditions, even if the inflammation reaction per se is interrupted and prevented from completing its mission by the above noted medications, the pathogen remains undisturbed, at times indefinitely, and so do the associated reddening, swelling, pain and overheating. A condition has been attained that prevents complete healing from taking place. Unfortunately, this is just the same condition that allows the damage to remain and allows development of further damage.

Promotion of inflammation

According to the researchers, anyone who protests that the enzyme preparations are described as being anti-inflammatory, i.e. inflammation inhibiting, and therefore not much better either, has not yet grasped that the goal of frequently administering high doses of enzyme mixtures is the opposite of inflammation inhibition. They can be best regarded as inflammation *activators* and *regulators*. A completely opposing principle of action is being followed here.

The researchers postulate that enzyme preparations, and particularly the anti-inflammatory enzyme mixtures (the most frequently used enzyme combinations), are therefore not inflammation inhibitors, but rather inflammation security brigades in charge of activation, regulation and repair. Accordingly, the therapeutic enzymes promote mechanisms which aid in limiting the damage, in its rectification, and in the formation of new healthy tissue. They accelerate the progress of the inflammation necessary for the healing of the wound. On the one hand, this acceleration means that the work of damage control, damage repair and new tissue construction is carried out more forcefully, efficiently and precisely, and is thus completed all the sooner. On the other hand, it also means that there can be a temporary increase in the visual and sensory effects produced by the inflammation; more reddening, more swelling, more warmth, more pain. That is not bad, and it does not require additional, separate treatment. It is a sign that the body is functioning, that the rescue and repair teams are hard at work.

Afterall, an inflammation is nothing more or less than the magnificent response of the body to local tissue damage. It is a beneficial reaction aimed at maintaining life. To suppress it, to interfere with it, will sooner or later result in some degree of bodily harm.

Thus, the scientists postulate that the therapeutic enzymes can better contribute to the proper activation and regulation of the immune defenses since they close the gap left from insufficient endogenous enzymes. They feel that it is no wonder enzyme mixtures can be used successfully to treat different disorders. The principle of an inflammatory reaction after a damaging stimulus plays an important role in combating the cause of almost every disorder known. For this reason, there is no need to continue with a complete description of all the disorders which have been treated by the application of this principle of inflammation assistance with the aid of enzyme mixtures.

Medical terminology makes use of the suffix 'itis' to describe many disorders involving inflammation; arthritis, pancreatitis, dermatitis, prostatitis, etc. Adnexitis, for instance, the inflammation of the fallopian tubes and surrounding tissues, according to the various researchers, incidentally responds excellently to treatment with the anti-inflammatory enzyme mixtures. This, they feel, expedites the resolution of the pathological or 'bad' inflammation. They also feel that many other disorders associated with acute or chronic inflammations can also be treated with enzyme mixtures.

We come back to the further possibilities for the use of systemic enzyme therapy for various disorders. In the same way, we return time and again to the effects of enzyme mixtures on immune processes. There are, in fact, two important basic mechanisms coming into action every time our health suffers. To better understand these, it is worth discussing injuries of all types, ranging from sports injuries to operations. In other words; the topic is the role of enzymes in traumatology.

Chapter 13

Injuries: Preparation is the key to it all

What is the most frequent health problem? A folk disease like rheumatism? No. Influenza? No. Well then, the common cold! Wrong again. The most frequent cause of ill health – as you might guess from the title of this chapter – is the common injury. The cut finger, the bump on the head, the bang on the knee, the twisted ankle or the simple bruise which you get because you walked into the corner of that damned cupboard again, or did not manage to fend off your lover.

And anyone who reads the chapter as well as its title will discover that every injury gives the alarm for an immediate rescue and repair service that involves numerous enzymes capable of the most varied tasks, the process of inflammation.

Our readers know that wherever anything is injured, the healing depends, to a very large extent, on the availability of increased quantities of the necessary endogenous enzymes at the site of injury. If everything is in order and sufficient enzymes arrive at the site of injury, the prospects are excellent that the wound will heal, the pain will die away and the whole story will soon be forgotten. This can be quite welcome whether it involves a twisted ankle or a tell-tale hickey.

Hickeys and karate blows

The enzymatic treatment of hickeys, or rather of bruises and hematomas, has been subjected to scientific investigation. However, the damage did not occur in such a pleasant manner, possibly to the disappointment of some of the hundred test subjects of both sexes who took part in the tests.

The investigation was carried out by two physicians in Germany of the Sports Medicine Investigation Center in Grünwald outside of Munich which is very well-known to German athletes. The physicians removed two cubic centimeters of blood from the antecubital vein of each subject and injected it just under the skin of the inside of the right forearm. This created a typical bruise in each of the subjects, a hematoma, as such a bruise is known medically (Figure 33).

Half of the subjects took 10 tablets of the anti-inflammatory enzyme mixtures three times daily, the others were 'treated' with placebo tablets containing no active components. The results were checked and measured daily; the amount of pain, how much pain was caused by pressure on the hematoma and how rapidly the hematoma disappeared.

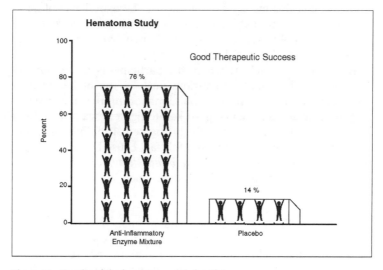

Figure 33: Results of the hematoma study by Kleine

The findings were convincing. The success rate was evaluated as 'good' by 76% of the anti-inflammatory enzyme mixture-treated subjects, and by only 14% of the placebo-treated subjects. The subjects treated with the anti-inflammatory enzyme mixtures felt less pain upon pressure, the pain caused by pressure disappeared more readily, and the visible hematoma disappeared much sooner.

It is no accident that sports physicians devised and carried out this experiment, since everyday injuries are accepted as quite normal consequences of virtually every sport, and their rapid healing is a challenge to every athlete, whether the aim is winning, a top performance, or simply the fun of competing.

There is little difference between the hickeys of a girl in love and a boxer's black eye. It is unimportant whether a football player is injured by collision with an opponent or an elderly man is injured when he slips on an icy sidewalk. The authors of the study felt that this means we can transfer the experience of treating sport injuries to daily injuries in the home or at work. Therefore, you should not be surprised when we report on an investigation involving 20 karate fighters.

Karate is a martial art where the participants try as hard as possible to deliver blows to various parts of the bodies of their opponents. There is no need to wait long for injuries to appear.

The investigation involving 20 karate fighters was carried out by Dr. Zuschlag – coincidentally, his name can be interpreted in German as meaning a 'strike', and this fact caused more comment than the actual results of a *double-blind study*, a study in which neither the physician nor the patient knew whether the anti-inflammatory enzyme mixtures or an inert substitute (placebo) were being taken (Figure 34).

Ten karate fighters, both men and women, were treated prophylactically with five of the anti-inflammatory enzyme tablets three times daily before fighting. The remaining ten received five tablets with no active components (placebo) three times daily. The severity of injuries suffered by the fighters was comparable for all 20 athletes.

At the end of the investigation, the distribution code was disclosed and the data were analyzed statistically. The results were

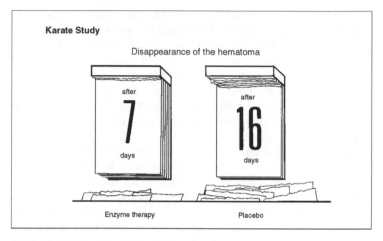

Figure 34: Results of the karate study

impressive: The athletes treated prophylactically with enzymes suffered hematomas which disappeared within 7 days; in the case of the athletes receiving no enzymes, this took 16 days (Figure 34). The swelling suffered by those in the enzyme-treated group had already subsided after a good four days, whereas those of the placebo group required ten days. Restrictions of movement as a result of pain and injury were absent after five days in the enzyme group, but lasted more than twelve days in the placebo group. When the injuries suffered during the karate fighting became inflamed, they had subsided after only four days in the former, but required eleven days to do so in the latter group.

In other words, the study concluded that when there is a risk of injury, it is possible to obtain some protection by taking an enzyme mixture prophylactically, and that the injuries actually being suffered cleared up in half or even one third of the time that it took if this precaution was not taken.

As already mentioned, the researchers felt that the results of this study can be extended to everyday life without any modifications. It does not matter whether you are an athlete or not. Similar double-blind studies have been carried out on the influence of the enzyme preparation on the subsidence of swelling and the healing of sprained ankles. This type of ankle injury is extremely common and certainly something which must have happened at least once to every nonathlete, and has remained in painful memory.

Reportedly, these and multiple other studies conclude that taking large quantities of enzyme tablets as soon as possible after an injury can lead to considerably quicker healing of the injury – with all the signs of a successfully terminated inflammatory process, that is with reduction of swelling, with diminishing pain, the restoration of free mobility and healthy tissue. They postulated that taking these enzymes prophylactically could therefore limit the extent of an injury and accelerate healing even more. All this is without the risk of serious side effects or the need for narcotics, and without the danger to an athlete of being accused of doping.

Only the healthy can win

If these enzyme preparations have this remarkable effect of protecting athletes from severe injury and making injuries heal faster, thus making him or her fit for the battle for points, goals, centimeters and fractions of a second, then coaches should consider having their athletes take them regularly.

In fact, according to some European Sports Medicine reports, there is scarcely a top athlete in Germany who is not familiar with the enzyme prophylaxis. Reportedly, "medical gurus of the big soccer, handball and ice hockey teams have them in their bags and distribute them generously before decisive matches." From Dr. Hans W. Müller-Wohlfahrt, the club doctor of the Bavarian Football Club, to such professors of Sports Colleges as Professor Klümper, to many other medical advisers for professional and top athletes, they recommend the protective and healing effects of the enzyme preparations.

Advocates of enzymes for sports injuries indicate that, although the type and extent of the injuries varies so much, the positive effects are confirmed again and again. Two of the sports physicians who were assigned to care for the German Olympic teams carried out a controlled investigation and obtained 'very good' to 'good' success rates in 82% of the athletes under their care, and that with the relatively low dose rate of only two tablets three times daily or even just three tablets daily. They were athletes who had suffered contusions, distortions, rupture of a capsule or ligament, edemas, hematomas, hydrarthroses, pulled or torn muscles, vertebral subluxations and other injuries falling within the description 'acute or chronic traumatic inflammations'. It goes without saying that the common 'tennis elbow' belongs to this category as well.

The Enzyme Research Institute suggests that scarcely an international sporting event takes place without some of the active participants using enzyme preparations. "This applies to world championships in soccer, handball and ice hockey, and the rather brutal American football, all sports where the risks of injury to the participants are high. It applies to the University championships in both the summer and winter sporting events. It applies to the admirable athletes competing in the Olympic Games for the handicapped."

At the Summer and Winter Olympics, sports physicians of several nations regularly contact the Enzyme Research Institute to obtain further scientific documentation regarding oral enzyme use in sports injuries.

For instance, the top Austrian athletes – runners, wrestlers, judokas, boxers, handball players, downhill skiers – were provided with the tablets as a prophylaxis against injury. One small example reported by Dr. Engel of the University Orthopedic Clinic of Vienna, will demonstrate their results with oral enzymes in the prophylaxis of sports injuries. He reported that, "although ten athletes without enzyme prophylaxis suffered injuries requiring suspension of sporting activities during the course of preparations for the games, there was only one athlete who was unable to compete fully on account of injury under the protection of enzyme prophylaxis during the actual competition. In all other cases of soft-tissue injuries, the dosage of enzymes was immediately increased, causing hematoma formation and soft-tissue inflammation to be rapidly and appreciably reduced so that the injured athletes were able to continue competing."

Professor Raas of the University of Innsbruck who is responsible for the Austrian athletes of the Winter Olympic games also confirmed these findings. He expressed the opinion that, "a good portion of the success achieved by the athletes under his care would not have been possible without enzyme preparations."

You are probably not one of the people intending to take part in the next Summer or Winter Olympics, but this does not diminish the importance of enzymes to us all. According to the Enzyme Research Institute, "in addition to the helpful effects of enzymes as prophylactic protection against normal everyday injuries, and as healing promoters after everyday injury, enzymes can also have another important personal aspect for you, namely, in the event of an operation."

An operation is a deliberate injury

Every operation is, among other things, a deliberately inflicted injury leading to acute inflammation. Every operation produces a wound, damages tissue, destroys blood vessels and warns our system that it must limit, clean-up and repair the damage.

Therefore, the Enzyme Research Institute recommends that, if there are no bleeding disorders, "enzymes should be taken before and after the operation in order to promote these important activities." They also stated that, "this is a very sensible method which only has limitations in cases of coagulation defects. In the latter, the steady state of blood flow is so out of balance that the enzymes might keep the blood too liquid. Inadequate blood clotting may not function as it should and this may interfere with wound closure."

Let us consider as an example an operation following injury to the meniscus of the knee joint. The torn, damaged meniscus must be removed, but the whole region around the knee joint is quite swollen as a result of the injury. This swelling is the result of a natural process, indeed, of a process required urgently in the course of any inflammation. The surgeon is now confronted with a new problem of removing the defective meniscus as rapidly as possible, since this operation is made more difficult by the misshapen swelling of the surrounding tissue. He would, therefore, be happy if the swelling would disappear as quickly as possible. According to some European orthopedic surgeons, the enzyme mixtures bring that about in a splendid manner.

After the operation to remove the meniscus, the physician remains quite concerned about the inflammation. The patient as well, who also finds the long wait for healing of the operative wound to be quite bothersome. After the operation, and with every day that passes, it still remains nearly impossible to move the knee joint on account of the further swelling caused by the surgical intervention, and the pain. In addition, if recovery is too slow or prolonged, the risk increases that the groups of muscles involved in joint function will atrophy. In earlier days when the healing took a longer period of time and the knee or half the leg was simply put into plaster, the result of the operation was often a stiff leg because it was not possible to promptly reactivate the knee joint.

Reports from double-blind studies in Wiesbaden by *Dr. Rahn*, an orthopedic surgeon, have indicated that the use of enzymes before and after meniscus operations brings both the physician and the patient considerable advantages (Figure 35).

For this reason, they and other surgeons suggest that it is sensible to administer enzymes both before and after the operative treatment of broken bones. It has been reported that patients who have been pretreated with enzymes are ready for operation 17 days after suffering broken bones since the edema subsides more rapidly, while patients not treated with enzymes were only operable after 24 days. The story was similar after surgery. While the patients with broken bones who had not been treated with enzymes required hospitalization for an average of 14 days before they could be discharged, those treated with enzymes were able to leave the clinic after only eight days.

The Enzyme Research Institute reviewed this and other studies and concluded that, "the period of confinement to bed is shortened both before and after surgery, there is also a reduction in the risk of thrombosis, an improvement in the mental state of the patient, a more rapid diminution of pain, a better and clearer operative site, more rapid healing of the wound with a healthier scar and, last but not least, appreciable savings in costs."

They also report that, "At present, operations are being undertaken in a number of European centers where the full range of enzyme action is exploited both before and after the surgical intervention, and that it is possible to call on the aid of the enzymes during surgery for some operations. Breast cancer operations are a case in point."

As already mentioned in the chapter describing the properties of enzymes, the surgeon naturally has to take into account the fibrin-degrading effects of enzymes in cases with increased risks of hemorrhage.

Enzymes, they feel, can even perform a useful function in operations to rectify blocked arteries. In operations of this type, the surrounding tissue can become involved in such a severe inflammatory reaction and thereby to such an extent that the vessel made patent by operative intervention can promptly be compressed and obstructed due to the pressure. The operation is therefore a failure and nothing has been gained. However, if the patient is subjected to preoperational enzyme treatment, it is possible to control the undesirable inflammatory swelling. The surgically opened arteries are no longer squashed and remain patent.

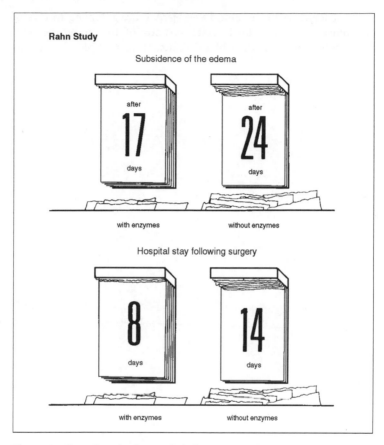

Rahn Study

Subsidence of the edema

after
17
days

after
24
days

with enzymes

without enzymes

Hospital stay following surgery

8
days

14
days

with enzymes

without enzymes

Figure 35: Above: Examination results before removal of meniscus
Below: Examination results after removal of meniscus

Professor *H. Denck*, a leading vascular surgeon in Vienna "has not been confronted with a single squashed artery since he began with this prophylactic measure."

That leads us to the blood vessels; we are referring to one of the most important steady state systems of the body, the very labile interaction between blood liquefaction and blood coagulation.

Chapter 14

The vessels: Everything flows

Immeasurable in its performance, immeasurable in its extent, our vascular system is a marvel; one that fills even the most experienced physicians with wonder.

We can only guess the total length of the interconnecting network of blood and lymph vessels, a million kilometers has been estimated. The tubes in these systems range from those as thick as your thumb to those which are so very fine that they can only be recognized under the microscope.

The blood vessels constantly transport from four to six liters of blood which, enriched with oxygen in the lesser pulmonary circulation, is pumped forcibly by the heart through the ever narrower arteries into the capillaries, thus supplying every single cell. The fine capillaries are so narrow that each minute cell in the bloodstream has to barely squeeze itself through. Once the capillaries have been traversed, the return flow begins through larger and ever larger veins, equipped with leaf valves. This is the difficult route back to the heart and the lungs which must be taken almost without pumping assistance from the heart, even though this pathway toward the heart is mainly uphill and against gravity.

This incredibly complicated cannular, pumping, suction and valvular system is a work of genius. It normally functions extremely well if, and this is the problem, the blood that it transports flows correctly.

Just like everything else in life or technology, it is all a question of the interchange between zero and one, between plus and minus or between yes and no; in the case of blood too there is a continual interaction and balance between solidity and fluidity, between coagulation and liquefaction. Blood has to be maintained in the correct state of fluidity in order to be able to nourish all the cells of the body and to transport away the metabolic wastes.

However, if the blood always stayed so fluid, it would be impossible for us to live, since the smallest injury to the giant network of vessels, a grazed knee, a cut finger, bleeding of the gums, would inevitably cause our blood to pour out at this point so that we would bleed to death. The wonderful capability of our blood to clot saves us from this fate. If it loses its state of fluidity, it becomes thicker and stickier and finally coagulates.

The glue which our blood produces for this purpose is known as *fibrin*. We require this fibrin not just to seal off wounds; it also acts continuously to coat the inner walls of the blood vessels with a thin layer which protects the delicate inner wall from damage by particles flowing within the vessel. The fibrin also makes good any small unevenness of the vascular wall so that the blood can flow without the formation of any disturbing eddies.

The body produces about 2 grams of fibrin daily for this purpose. Accordingly, if not properly regulated, the walls of our blood vessels might be expected to gradually become coated by a thickening layer of this adhesive material so that the vessels become less and less permeable and finally no more blood can flow through them.

Fortunately, we do not just possess a system for the production of adhesive fibrin, but also have a cleverly controlled system for continual fibrin dissolution. The purpose of this is to degrade excess fibrin formation and thus maintain a steady state of blood flow.

This continual struggle for an equilibrium between blood coagulation and blood liquefaction, so-called *fibrinolysis*, is one of the most important factors in the maintenance of a person's health. (Figures 36 and 37). If fibrinolysis increases too much, the blood becomes too thin and there is a danger of bleeding to death, the danger of becoming a bleeder, such as in a condition also known as hemophilia. Too much fibrin production, where the blood becomes too thick and sticky, is a much more common condition.

This stickiness of the blood as a result of overproduction of fibrin, or an insufficient rate of its breakdown, is the most frequent accompanying symptom of the disorders which are more fatal than all others, diseases of the cardiovascular system.

It should be pointed out, as mentioned in the sections dealing with rheumatoid arthritis and multiple sclerosis, that fibrin is important in reference to our immune defenses since it also forms an important layer or mantle around the tissue-bound immune complexes, which although intended to protect us at these sites, also hinders by limiting the other immune defenses.

Never too much and never too little

On account of its central importance, we will now digress to a brief discussion of how the steady state of blood flow functions. This process is fascinating for everyone (Figures 36 and 37).

The task being considered is by no means easy for the body to carry out. It has to ensure that the flow properties of the blood are optimal and, at the same time, be on the alert to drive the equilibrium in one particular direction in any part of the body. This equilibrium is kept in balance through the action of several naturally occurring enzymes in the blood system that interact with each other in a fascinating fashion. Let's start with *fibrin*, the glue. In an emergency, fibrin is needed immediately, and the body cannot allow itself too much time to make it from scratch to seal off a wound. On the other hand, the adhesive must not be activated unnecessarily and stop the flow of blood in the wrong area.

The adhesive is therefore found everywhere in the bloodstream, but not in its active, sticky form; not in the form of fibrin itself, but as its precursor, another enzyme form named *fibrinogen*. Fibrinogen has a thin threadlike structure made up of a chain of either *five or eight protein molecules* attached to one another. There are millions of such molecules of fibrinogen floating in the blood serum, in the plasma, and they have no tendency whatsoever to accumulate anywhere. Fibrinogen does not do anything, it is harmless, it is another weapon with a very secure safety catch.

Only at the moment the safety catch is removed does the fibrinogen become active. This safety catch is merely a single link of the protein chain so that the chain is afterwards only made up of either *four or seven members* (Figure 36). This immediately causes fibrinogen to lose its previous stability, it attaches itself to a neighboring fibrinogen which has also lost its stability and they clump together to form the adhesive fibrin.

A very simple principle, one member is pinched off each protein chain and the blood at that site clots where it is needed, for instance to seal off a wound. When the clot is exposed to air it loses moisture and dries, in a sort of dry, shrunken layer, to form a hard protective scab.

This thing that removes a chain link from the stable fibrinogen, turning it into the clot-forming fibrin, is naturally one of the protein-cleaving enzymes. This enzyme is called *thrombin* and its purpose is to produce fibrin in order to cause blood to thicken and to coagulate on command (Figure 37). Like all enzymes, thrombin carries out this activity rather unimaginatively and automatically without taking into account whether the result is useful or not. This risk, which applies to every enzyme activity, is the reason the whole enzyme process has to be accompanied by complicated safety devices; with the accompanying disadvantage that errors can at times occur in the system.

Thus, for the sake of safety, this fibrin-producing enzyme *thrombin* (Figure 37) is not present in the blood serum in the active form, but, just like fibrinogen, in an inactive precursor form, as *prothrombin*. Should the alarm be sounded, a whole series of consecutive reactions catalyzed by about twelve different enzymes is triggered off as quick as a flash. The final result is an activator for converting the sleeping prothrombin into 'ready-for-anything' thrombin. The activator acts rather like the second arm of a pair of tweezers. One-armed tweezers are no good for anything, but once the second arm is present, thrombin can function. It nips off the safety catch of fibrinogen and turns it into sticky fibrin.

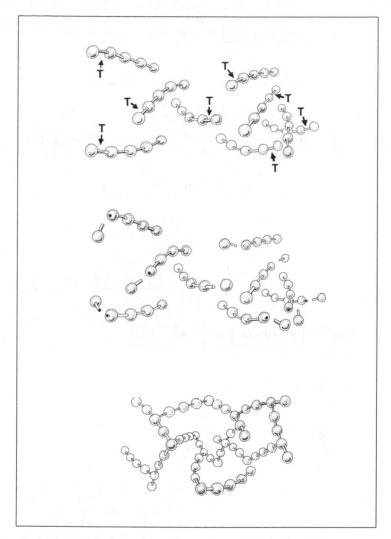

Figure 36: Fibrin formation: Thrombin (T) removes individual links from the fibrinogen chain which then bind to form a network

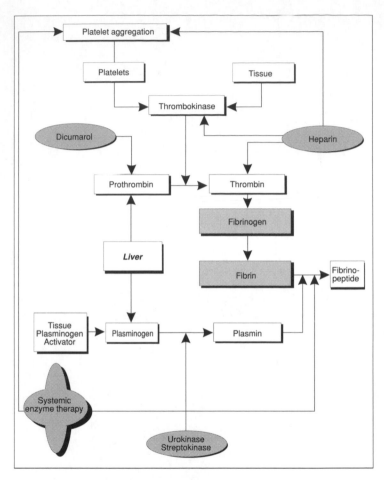

Figure 37: Schematic representation of coagulation and fibrinolysis pathways illustrating sites of action of anticoagulants and postulated sites of action of
systemic oral enzyme therapy. Fibrinolysis (shaded area) results in the
release of fibrinopeptides which can be reused as building blocks

Everything flows again with plasmin

There is never a no without a yes, a plus without a minus, a function without a counterfunction. For this reason, we must have a system for re-liquefying the sticky blood, that is for dissolving the sticky adhesive fibrin, and therefore the associated clot, for so-called *fibrinolysis* (Figure 37). That also occurs according to the frugal laws of nature; when a clever and simple principle has been developed it should be upheld and exploited in every way possible.

Fibrinolysis also proceeds according to the principle of activation of previously protected inactive enzymes. Blood serum therefore contains another harmless, inactive proenzyme with a safety catch on, namely *plasminogen*. It too is activated when needed by means of numerous, varied enzymes acting one after the other and finally serving to convert the inert plasminogen into active *plasmin*.

Plasmin chops off individual members of the giant protein molecule of fibrin, causing the fibrin to degrade into separate stable protein chains which can be transported away. Easy come, easy go; thrombin nips off a bit of a soluble protein molecule and an adhesive results, plasmin nips off a bit of the adhesive and it once again dissolves.

Fibrinolysis is a nice example of how nature chooses the best technique every time, or almost everytime. However, nature is not immune from errors in the system. The particular danger here is if the dissolution of fibrin and clots does not take place because of an error in plasmin activation. If fibrinolysis does not occur, we have serious blood flow problems in the arteries and veins. In addition, we have problems at other sites where fibrin is also required and deposited. Thus, inadequate fibrinolysis can also lead to the blockage of the ducts of the lacrimal, salivary and mammary glands, and the ureters would not remain open. Fibrinolysis also plays an important role in the bleeding during menstrual periods. Furthermore, if fibrinolysis failed, the liver, kidneys and lungs would also become brawn-like and harden, and finally all organs would simply cease to function.

A further complication is that fibrinolysis takes place at different rates in different parts of our bodies. Thus, the fibrin-dissolving activity in the veins is higher than it is in the arteries, and it is higher in the veins of the arm than it is in the veins of the leg. This is a result of differences in the plasmin levels, that is the amount and quality of plasmin to be found in each of the different regions. Plasmin alone is capable of degrading the sticky fibrin into its components.

Plasmin levels generally sink with increasing age. At 60, we only possess a fraction of the plasmin which we had when young. We know the results; the blood flows more sluggishly, toxic debris tends to remain in the vessels, the vessels become narrower due to deposits, and they harden. Disturbances occur which tend to aggravate one another until disease results; insufficient blood flow to the heart, the brain and the legs as far as varicose veins, and other symptoms which are virtually accepted as the normal state of affairs in the elderly.

Thrombi, cholesterol and other dangers

Plasmin activation has already been described in the section on "faithful servants" and the attentive reader will perhaps remember that this plasmin did not only dissolve fibrin, but was also the means for the dissolution of blood clots. This is not particularly surprising since clots, also called thrombi, normally consist of fibrin and the substances deposited in this fibrin.

What happens is illuminating; when the blood is too sticky, the danger exists that small clots form and can then be deposited at the next bend of the blood vessel or in a narrower vessel. A barrier at which the next little blood clot can be deposited is then formed until, in the end, blood can no longer flow past.

Plasmin activation to dissolve fibrin is thus a decisive measure to combat the danger of disturbances to the flow of blood in the veins and arteries. The most gentle way of promoting the dissolution of fibrin and clots by a drug is undoubtedly the systemic administration of fibrinolytic enzymes. European reports postulate that this also applies to the enzyme mixtures which contain the 'faithful servants' required for plasmin activation.

According to the Enzyme Research Institute, this has been demonstrated in countless double-blind studies. They have reported that such oral enzyme mixtures are able to dissolve the little clots which are referred to as microthrombi and are able to normalize the blood-flow equilibrium. They postulate that, "the oral enzyme mixtures can exert a positive effect on the tendency of blood platelets to clump and harden, the blood can be freed from metabolic wastes; order and normality can be restored."

Some degree of fibrinolysis is constantly necessary, our blood-flow is continuously under attack. Not just from microthrombi, excess cholesterol is involved as well. Cholesterol stands accused as the principal culprit in all cardiovascular diseases, but it is basically a vitally important component of cell membranes and a starting material for many hormones. It is a fatty substance which we ourselves produce and which we additionally take in with our food.

A cholesterol deficiency can injure your health, but the concentration of cholesterol in the blood is usually too high. The Europeans also postulate that the enzyme mixture makes it possible to lower the blood concentration of cholesterol and also that of triglycerides. Triglycerides are the body's biggest energy store and found particularly in fatty tissue. They are essential to a point, but excesses are harmful. We are therefore obliged to eat and live more sensibly.

The danger which is caused by the cholesterol floating around in the blood does not lie in the fact that it is a fatty substance which glues up our vessels like fat sticking to a pan, but instead, it takes a form that is not normally thought of as 'fat'. The cholesterol takes the form of *pointed crystals*. When the blood pressure is high and the blood contains many of these pointed crystals of cholesterol, they are pressed into the walls of the vessel. That particular portion of the vessel then loses its elasticity and becomes covered with a deposit. Special phagocytic cells (histiocytes) come to this site where they form a cluster of cells and attempt to clear these deposits and eliminate the crystals. Together they constitute a cholesterol plaque. The hindrance to flow brings about further disturbances and the vicious cycle continues. This is the start of arteriosclerosis.

The pointed cholesterol crystals lead to a further danger. It has been postulated in the medical literature that the vessel walls damaged by the crystals change their structure in such a manner that our immune systems mistakenly assume the damaged vessel walls are not part of the body but rather foreign material which must be combated and removed. Thus, the medical literature speaks of the vessel walls possessing an 'antigenic effect' which mobilizes the body's defenses against foreign bodies. The body fights against itself in this way and we suffer from an autoaggressive disorder.

This always involves inflammation and other changes that mislead the immune system. There are numerous immunologically based vascular disorders. In this manner, such diseases resulting from the body's defenses being misled, such as chronic rheumatoid arthritis or lupus erythematosus, can themselves extend to the entire vascular system and bring about inflammation in all layers of the vessel walls. A so-called *vasculitis* results.

Since it has already been discussed several times how every inflammatory disorder and every disorder resulting from immune complexes can be improved by optimizing the enzyme availability, no one will be surprised to discover that enzyme mixtures have also been used in the treatment of vasculitis. This has been reported in many publications. The most common publications regarding the administration of enzyme mixtures for cardiovascular disorders concern the investigations on chronic disorders of the veins.

Leg ailments, much ado about nothing?

Vein illnesses? So what? Even the occasional physician will say that nearly everyone suffers from this, and that it is only a trifling matter. Insignificant, it is not! About 59% of ordinary people suffer from this malady. This means that 147.5 million of the 250 million population in the United States, or 47 million of the 80 million citizens of the unified Germany, particularly between 20 and 70 years of age, suffer from some complaints involving the veins. Fifteen percent have varicose veins in an advanced stage, meaning 37.5 million in the U.S. and 12 million people in unified Germany. About 12% suffer from chronic complaints of the veins, that is 30 million in the U.S. and 9.6 million in unified Germany alone.

There are naturally disorders of the veins which are not particularly dramatic such as the supposedly harmless, 'sunburst' small varicose dilations of the cutaneous veins which are the first precursors of true varicose veins. However, the conditions can progress, enlarge and deteriorate to form blood clots or deep vein thromboses. The first danger associated with venous thrombosis is that it can possibly result in small detached blood clots that move inside the veins towards the heart or may lead to pulmonary or other embolisms. This is a serious medical condition and can result in death if unattended. About 152,000 people in the United States and 49,000 in unified Germany die as a consequence of the various venous diseases and their complications each year. Let us look in more detail into these problems.

Unfortunately, the naming of venous disorders is as chaotic as that of the rheumatic group of diseases. They are perhaps best classified under the heading "'chronic venous insufficiency'.

Chronic venous insufficiency makes itself felt as pain which is sometimes burning and sometimes penetrating, and primarily found at night. The legs feel alternately hot and cold, standing for long periods is not possible without fatigue, the ankles swell. The unsightliness of varicose veins is not their only problem, the poor circulation becomes more and more of a handicap whether sitting, standing or walking. Eventually, the insufficiency fails to remove metabolites and toxins and the skin of the lower legs begins to starve for nutrients. Chronic skin insufficiency ('stasis dermatitis') also results and this can lead to the dreaded and painful chronic leg ulcers. The problem is often associated with deep venous thrombosis (clots) and followed by increased venous insufficiency.

Every shop assistant knows that the poor old veins were simply never intended to transport blood against gravity from the feet to the heart. That was something our ancestors did not take properly into account as they climbed down from the trees and began their careers as the upright, two-legged forerunners of civilization.

We now have to put up with this inappropriate design. We can give the veins in our legs some help if we gently massage our ankles and calves every day, frequently stand on tiptoe or simply put up our feet like cowboys, but that will not protect our veins completely from damage. The formation of thrombi by blood which is too sluggish is the start of many venous disorders.

Surely, you can try to remove the clots, even going as far as surgery, but the thrombi unfortunately settle too frequently in the veins and can no longer be broken down and transported away no matter how many enzymes are taken. The vein has become blocked, a dead end is formed.

The blood has to find another route. New venous routes are formed as a detour so that the venous blood can still reach the heart, but the thrombus in the blocked vein still constitutes a danger. Afterall, the venous blood still pressing against the thrombus usually continues to bring microthrombi with it which can be deposited in the same region of the legs, and make this focus of poor health grow and grow.

It is therefore absolutely necessary to promote breakdown of the microthrombi as well to normalize the equilibrium of blood consistency. The answer here is again clear, remove and prevent the clots! Conservative medical treatment of these deep venous clots generally required anticoagulants. However, more and more frequently, the acute venous thrombosis process is treated with intravascular enzymatic thrombolysis as discussed in the introduction. The Enzyme Research Institute strongly advocates the administration of sufficient active enzymes in the required amount and quality for both prevention and treatment.

The second danger associated with venous thrombosis is a result of the high degree of pressure in front of the blockage. This pressure enlarges the vessel, causing large protein molecules to be forced into the surrounding tissue and to take plasma fluid with them. Edema results and is seen as 'swollen legs'.

Initially, this is just a cosmetic problem as far as most people are concerned, but the state of health in the legs is far more important than their appearance, since the proteins which escape from the veins before the obstructions change to such an extent that they are treated as foreign substances and attacked. The connective tissue cells around the congested and blocked vessels are stimulated to grow, the region becomes indurated (hardened), lymph vessels are also compressed and cause lymphedema in the tissues as well, further increasing the swelling.

The fact that inflammatory processes now take place in the affected region can be seen from the typical symptoms which are always indicative of an inflammation; pain, warmth, swelling, reddening. Because the veins are affected, the acute inflammation is called phlebitis.

The inflammation taking place in the region surrounding the vein and before the blockage leads, among other things, to an activation of fibrin, since signals are sent out to the body that there is an injury which must be dealt with. This intensifies the production of fibrin which was initially already part of the cause of the entire problem.

It is in this manner that the disease amplifies itself, it is self-perpetuating, as the physicians are fond of saying. This condition is known as a *post-thrombotic syndrome*, that is the state after thrombosis. The conventional medical view is that there is not an awful lot that can be done about it. It is certainly helpful to wear an elastic support stocking, but it must be the correct one that is fitted properly and worn continually. Unfortunately, not many people with venous disorders are willing to wear such a stocking. At least 60% of patients who are advised to wear an elastic stocking refuse to do so or just leave it in the drawer. There are also numerous therapeutic agents which have been used, but none have helped significantly or have offered a lasting effect. Even horse chestnut preparations have been proposed to offer relief, but treatment is far from adequate and that is all that can be done if conventional opinion is to be believed.

Demonstrable improvement

Physicians frustrated with the inadequacy of conventional medical treatment would doubtlessly be pleased to be able to find a better treatment. It is therefore worthwhile to review the European experience in this context. They report the results of multiple well-conducted investigations detailing remarkable success in the treatment of vein problems with oral enzyme therapy.

As early as 1962, Professor Dr. J. Valls-Serra, Director of the Department of Angiology and Vascular Surgery of the University of Barcelona, Spain published his experiences with the enzyme treatment of venous inflammation, "Our therapeutic results are excellent, particularly with respect to the duration of therapy. In the case of earlier methods of treatment, it took several months for severe phlebitides (venous inflammations) to heal. The present methods of treatment bring about healing within only a few weeks. However, for postphlebitic syndrome as well, that is the continuance of symptoms six months after the appearance of the primary phlebitis, the results were also astonishingly good and superior to all methods of vessel dilation and anticoagulant therapy previously undertaken."

In the U.S., in 1972, Professor Wolf reported the results of treating 347 patients with venous disorders of various types using the enzyme mixture (Figure 38). Here, he observed that, "58% of patients suffering from superficial phlebitis were completely freed from all symptoms, a further 29% became almost free from symptoms. Only 13% exhibited no improvement or only a slight improvement. The length of time required for treatment was also considerably less than that in the control group. The improvement took place in one half to one third the time required in the case of the control group."

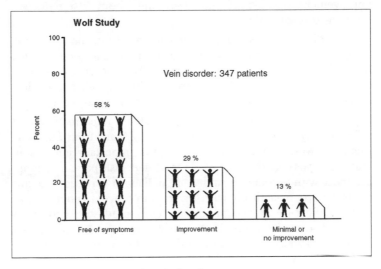

Figure 38: Results of therapy for vein disorders

Dr. H. Denck, Professor and Chairman of the Surgical Department of the Municipal Hospital of Vienna, has published similar results. A clinical study of the treatment of post-thrombotic syndrome by enzyme therapy revealed that 41% of the patients had been completely freed from the disorder or were vastly improved after eight weeks, 53% were very much better, whereas 6% reported no change in their condition (Figure 39).

Naturally, the treatment of vein disorders with enzyme therapy does not have to be restricted to hospitals. In order to collect the experiences of general practitioners, Dr. Maehder carried out a multicenter study on their patients. An analysis was made of the results of treating 216 cases of various vein disorders with enzymes. The study results indicated that 31% of the patients had completely recovered, after enzyme therapy and that there was an improvement in 62% of the cases and about 7% remained unchanged (Figure 39).

According to the various reports in the European literature, "enzyme therapy is not confined to those vein disorders which have already reached the chronic stage. The preventive value of this method of treatment is even greater, since it makes it possible to reduce the chances of these disorders occurring as we age."

Thus, in his publication on the oral enzyme treatment of inflammatory venous disorders, Dr. Herbert Mahr from Bad Dürrheim, in western Germany came to the important conclusion that, "it is possible to successfully treat high-risk patients (smokers, those with improper or imbalanced diets, or exposed to toxins or stress) prophylactically with enzymes to prevent venous disorders. In the case of occupations virtually predestined to suffer venous disorders (nurses, barbers, salesmen or housewives, all occupations which involve a great deal of standing), enzyme preparations can be administered to protect the circulation."

When you consider that up to 60% of the adult population of the United States or of Germany has vein trouble at least temporarily, that one in every eight adults suffers from chronic venous insufficiency, and that 12 million in the U.S. and over 2 million people in unified Germany suffer from nonhealing leg sores as a result of venous problems, you can imagine how important such prophylaxis is. One fact in particular emphasizes the importance of sensible and acceptable preventive treatment for those with a

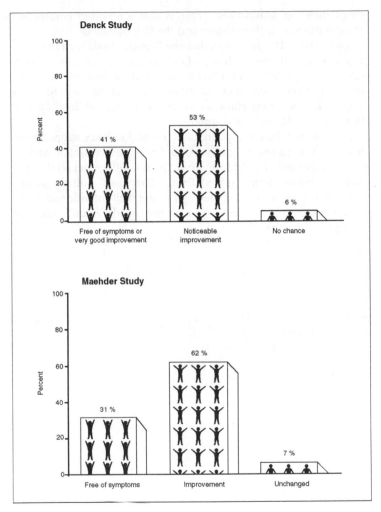

Figure 39: Above: Study results of patients with post-thrombotic syndrome
Below: Study results of patients with vein disorders

risk of suffering thrombosis. There is also a reported connection between the risk of thrombosis and the risk of cancer.

It was about 100 years ago that the French physician Trousseau drew attention to the tendency of cancer patients to suffer thromboses and of patients with thrombosis to suffer from cancer. Cancer researchers have since confirmed this, using, among other things, the dissection statistics of the Pathological Institutes in Hamburg and Munich in Germany.

The common factor appears fairly clear. Evidence supports the idea that the culprit is undissolved fibrin, under which and in which cancer cells can hide as under a camouflage net so that the body's defenses cannot get at them. They can multiply undisturbed and form a tumor. Once again, the well-intentioned fibrin mantle designed by nature to protect the health, actually ends up having the opposite effect.

Chapter 15

Cancer: The enemy we know

"He slaughtered lambs, he slaughtered piglets, he slaughtered calves. He removed the young animals' pancreases and minced them into small pieces, rinsed the pulp, filtered off the watery liquid and took it to his cancer patients." It is almost one-hundred years ago that the British embryologist John Beard began to treat what were thought to be incurable cancer patients in this highly unusual manner. He had devoted his life to a study of the processes leading to the production of an entire organism out of a fertilized egg in the body. He was convinced that every sort of growth, all further development of life, was intimately bound to enzyme activity, associated with those strange substances about which so little was known in those days. Nevertheless, one thing was known, important enzymes were principally produced in the pancreas. Beard reasoned that if a growth process got out of control, as is the case with cancer, this might be a result of a deficiency in these important enzymes necessary for every healthy development.

He was not entirely clear about this, but he developed an interesting theory and then went to work. His theory was borne out of practice. He believed that young animals ought to have the most powerful enzymes. Afterall, they need the most energy for growth. He therefore took pancreases of newborn lambs, pigs and calves, and pressed out the fluids containing concentrated enzymes. Very shortly after slaughter, he injected the fluid obtained from the filtered pancreatic juices slowly into the veins or the muscles of the buttocks in his cancer patients. Sometimes he injected it into the tumor itself if the tumor could be reached with a needle.

His treatments were not always successful. The unpurified juices also contained foreign proteins, and allergic reactions or even shock sometimes occurred. Dr. Beard's colleagues were of the opinion that this mad embryologist was a scandal to the medical profession and wanted to close down his practice. They pointed to the patients who had been in mortal danger on account of their allergic reactions. They referred to the patients who died of cancer in spite of his treatment.

Dr. Beard did not allow himself to be discouraged, since most of the patients who came to him were suffering from cancer in its terminal stages. He was prepared to try anything which promised even a ghost of a chance. Dr. Beard then experienced how the tumor masses actually disappeared under the influence of the injected enzymes, how cancer growth was inhibited, how numerous patients survived longer than had been prophesized.

He treated a total of 170 cancer patients in this manner. In 1907, he wrote a book, "The Enzyme Treatment of Cancer and its Scientific Basis" which was concerned with his experiences. In this book, he described how he was able to help more than half of the patients with advanced cancer using the pancreatic juices of newborn lambs, pigs and calves. How some cancers thought to be quite incurable completely disappeared, how patients recovered and their lives were prolonged.

This book caused a furor in England. His colleagues were naturally plagued by their cancer patients to treat them with this marvellous pancreatic juice with which Dr. Beard had had such great success. Why not? The physicians ordered filtered pancreatic juices from their pharmacists. The pharmacists in turn ordered the juices from the local slaughterhouse.

In this manner, however, Dr. Beard's colleagues administered inactive juices which were absolutely useless. Afterall, they were prepared from older animals. In addition, the enzymes had long since degraded themselves since enzymes are active in aqueous solution and have an active life which can be measured in hours. Dr. Beard, on the other hand, had used enzymatic juices prepared from young animals and administered these juices to the patients freshly after slaughter.

Since the physician's colleagues did not meet with success and bitterly disappointed their patients, Dr. Beard's method was quickly forgotten. Peace reigned once again in the medical profession and no one was forced to believe in the 'absurd theory that the embryologist had dreamed up'.

On the trail

Decades passed by before Dr. Max Wolf in his New York practice wrote to all archives of the western world asking them to send him all the information they could on 'cancer and enzymes'.

It was this same Professor Wolf whose story has already been told who got to know the Viennese physician Dr. Ernst Freund at the start of the 1930's. The Dr. Freund who, in collaboration with Dr. Kaminer, had published a short article with the unprepossessing title, "The Biochemical Basis of Disposition to Carcinoma".

In this article, Freund and Kaminer described how they had added blood serum of healthy subjects to cancer cells in cell cultures and had discovered that the serum must contain something which combated cancer; also that the blood of cancer sufferers did not contain this substance or that it was inhibited by a 'blocking factor'.

Professor Wolf decided to follow up this clue, isolate the mysterious substance and discover the blocking factor. It became more and more evident that the substance appeared to consist of enzymes.

He probably read everything that had been written or investigated about enzymes up to that time. He also read one of the few remaining copies of Dr. Beard's book moldering away in some scientific library or other. He thought he knew why Dr. Beard had been successful and his poor imitators had failed.

The result is history! At the start of the 1950's in his Biological Research Institute Laboratory at Columbia University, New York, Professor Wolf began an immensely complicated and difficult series of time-consuming tests. Together with his coworker Dr.

Helen Benitez, thousands of cell cultures were prepared in which cancer cells and normal cells grew together. These cell cultures were then treated with individual enzymes in order to discover which enzymes were particularly active in degrading the cancer cells while leaving healthy cells unaffected.

The whole range of enzymes was screened for those with the greatest potency and greatest safety, that is those which were only effective against malignant and not against healthy cells. Tests were then carried out to investigate which combination of enzymes yielded the greatest synergy, that is which mutually increased the activity to the greatest degree.

One of the enzyme preparations developed in this way was Wolf and Benitez's oncologic enzyme mixture, an agent which has been administered to about 50,000 cancer patients per year over the past 25 years in western Germany alone.

As a reaction to his work, Wolf initially received protest, skepticism or even derision from most traditionally-oriented physicians. Wolf and his coworkers were not treated very differently than the embryologist Dr. Beard.

According to his reports, the dreaded side effects, the allergic shock reactions, did not occur when the cancer patients were treated with the enzyme mixture, thanks to the high purity of these enzymes. It was possible to even maintain the activity of the enzymes in storage by stabilizing them and the uptake of the enzymes was considerably increased over the method of Dr. Beard by the use of simple physiological tricks. However, none of this deterred many traditional academic physicians from coming to a damaging conclusion, "Pure charlatanry!"

Today we forget too easily that it was established medical opinion 25 years ago that cancer was a local disorder. Professor K.H. Bauer, at the time President of the German Cancer Society, was prepared to call anyone who presumed there was a relationship between cancer and the body's immune system a charlatan.

It is true that our knowledge of the causes of cancer was by no means so advanced as it is today, it is also true that knowledge about the immune system was nearly nonexistent. However, as the years passed, the old attitudes were found to be more and more lacking and the justification for, among other things, the treatment of cancer, by means of enzyme mixtures, turned out to be a sound one.

Do not lose control

The reason why and how enzymes can have a favorable effect on the cancer process is relatively simple to understand, at least for those who have fought their way this far through the book and for whom the concept of immune complexes is no longer so exotic. But, first of all, how does cancer occur?

Cancer cells are formed under the influence of many different factors, as a result of physical, chemical, infectious, immunological and genetic mechanisms which interfere with the process of production of the body's cells. These influences, cause a tiny change in the structure of the cell leading to the production of a new protein which does not form part of the body's own cell structure, thus producing a deranged cell. It should also be pointed out that, according to some reports in the medical literature, one of the factors that may contribute to the abnormal cellular protein can also consist of a psychologically triggered nerve impulse.

The faulty, malformed cell thus becomes a cancer cell. The problem is that it is no longer subject to the body's control systems and is egotistic, only thinking of itself and only being subject to an urge to grow and multiply. To do this it robs the other cells and the body of precious nutrients. The good thing is that it is different from the normal cells of the body and can be recognized as foreign because of its foreign structure and, thus, it is subject, like any other foreign intruder, to being searched out, attacked and destroyed by the body's own defenses.

This construction error takes place relatively rarely, but with the billions of cells which are being produced within our bodies

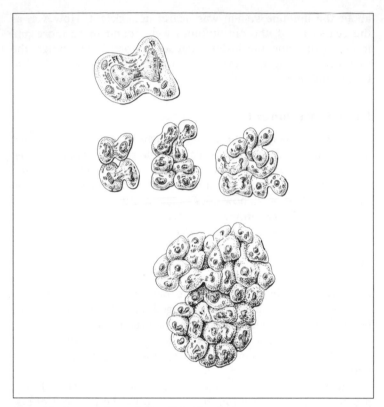

Figure 40: Cancer cell growth via cell division

during every minute of our lives, this means that every healthy person could have 100 to 10,000 such individual deranged or cancer-like cells in the body at any given moment (Figure 40). That is quite normal. It does not mean you are suffering from 'cancer' since the malformed, degenerate cells are continually recognized by our body's own intact defense systems and engulfed and eliminated by our predatory macrophages. Or they are attacked by our antibodies, signals for help are sent out and a killer group of suitable enzymes answers the call and disintegrates the cancer-like cell. The toxic debris which remains is finally transported away enzymatically.

The supervision functions as follows: New cancer-like cells are produced constantly, but about as many are recognized and destroyed. A few of these individual cancer-like cells survive, but they just float about aimlessly in the blood, they find nowhere to anchor themselves and die off of their own accord without having to be attacked by the immune system.

Things are more difficult when this balance is upset. For instance, outside influences cause many more faulty cells to be produced than usual. These influences – environmental pollution, poor living and eating habits, drugs that weaken the immune system, carcinogens in tobacco smoke, sunburn, radiation, loss of function that comes with advancing age – weaken our body's defenses to some degree.

All this causes the balance between friend and foe to be displaced. The weakened defenses can no longer hold the increased numbers of enemies in check. Now, cancer has its chance.

A significant number of the cancer cells now escape destruction. They can adhere to cell walls and multiply while in hiding. That is a particularly dangerous trick of cancer cells. They seem to know that our body's defenses can recognize them and destroy them because they are different. In order to avoid this, they coat themselves with the adhesive fibrin. The fibrin layer over cancer cells is about 15 times thicker than that of normal cells. They hide their suspicious markings, their antigens, under a layer of glue so that they are not recognized as enemies. Once again, the fibrin mantle causes trouble.

The sticky cancer cells can wander at will through the blood or lymph vessels. Because of their adhesiveness, they can get caught inside a blood clot, or on a bend or tiny bump of the vessel wall. Again they coat themselves with more fibrin and multiply under this camouflage. In this way, millions of cancer cells can accumulate in their hiding place to form a tumor, break through the vessel wall as they expand and penetrate further into the tissue.

The cancer cells can grow because of the absence of the enzymes that Freund and Kaminer looked for in the past, enzymes capable of stripping the fibrin from the individual cancer cells, laying bare their antigens and so paving the way for their destruction by macrophages and the whole might of the immune system. The more cancer cells the body produces, the more enzymes the body needs.

A dirty trick

Cancer cells have no inhibitions, they are egotistic and primitive. However, they are also clever, wily gangsters that are up to every trick to outwit the body's police force.

The cancer cells want to deter enzymes from tearing away their protective fibrin and alerting the immune system to their presence. Their aim is to block the enzymes and the immune system. Once established, in addition to the fibrin, there actually are certain 'blocking factors' that put our immune system pretty well out of action.

We now know what one of these 'blocking factors' is. We must return to our famous immune complexes in order to understand its action and why it is so important.

In theory, every cancer cell bears a specific antigen on its surface. Naturally, it is ideal when this tell-tale 'trademark', freed from fibrin, is recognized so that the cell can be destroyed. However, when the cancer cell is destroyed, the antigen can remain behind. In addition, the cancer cells sometimes succeed in modifying their membranes so that some of the antigens are released, apparently in order to trick our defense systems by leaving a false track. Also, new antigens are often formed.

Unfortunately, this dirty trick on the part of the cancer cells works. Our antibodies, the watchmen of our defenses, attack all antigens whether they sit on a cancer cell or float about alone.

This means that antibody-antigen complexes are constantly being produced, but unfortunately often with antigens that are no longer attached to cancer cells and therefore cannot lead to the cancer cell.

If the numbers of these immune complexes stay within limits, our defenses remain intact, since our macrophages succeed in engulfing and devouring the immune complexes. However, should the numbers of immune complexes exceed the capabilities of our macrophages, the undegraded immune complexes remain in the blood and the lymph.

A complex mechanism, we speak of *platelet activation and aggregation*, leads to increased fibrin formation when the undegraded immune complexes deposit themselves in the tissue. This would lower the defense forces under normal conditions, but is indeed particularly dangerous if the body is menaced by cancer.

As if all this were not enough, the surviving immune complexes also alarm and trigger the complement cascade, i.e. the interlinked chain of enzymes with the killer instinct. The actual target of this chain reaction is the destruction of such enemies as bacteria, viruses and cancer cells as well. However, the wildly firing complement cascade brings about inflammation and renewed tissue damage when it occurs, and is also connected with increased fibrin formation.

The immune complexes can also weaken the immune defenses in other ways. Too many immune complexes can inhibit the activity of the major destroyers of cancer cells, the macrophages. Their ability to devour and destroy is lost, the cancer cells can multiply without hindrance.

Many scientific investigations have concluded that the primary 'blocking factors' for cancer are immune complexes. Increased concentrations of immune complexes can be measured in the blood and lymph, and in the region of the tumor, in almost all important forms of human cancer. It is even possible to make predictions concerning the likely course of the disease; the higher the

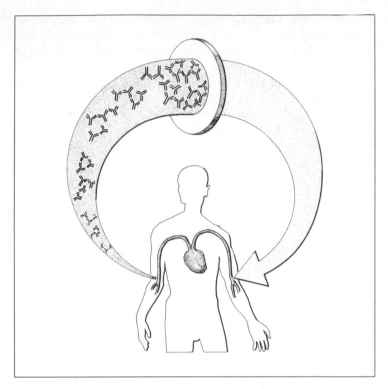

Figure 41: Simplified representation of plasmapheresis: Immune complexes are filtered from the blood; after its withdrawal, the 'purified' blood is then reinjected

concentration of circulating immune complexes, the lower the prospects of a favorable course for the disease.

Naturally, these recent results concerning defense inhibition as a result of too many immune complexes have resulted in attempts to filter the damaging immune complexes out of the blood and plasma of cancer patients. This can be performed by means of new techniques called plasmapheresis or lymphapheresis (Figure 41) where the blood and lymph is led out of the patient, mechanically separated from the immune complexes and then returned to the patient's body. Cryoprecipitation (precipitation brought about by cooling) takes place in a similar manner while the use of protein A causes the immune complexes to adhere to this specific protein. There have already been some encouraging successes in the treatment of cancer using these measures, particularly in the United States.

Illness protects against cancer

Nowhere on earth have more mental effort and money been expended in the search for factors and substances that can bring about or inhibit cancer than in the United States.

One of the undoubted leaders in the field is the Sloan-Kettering Institute in New York where Professor Lloyd Old was active for many decades. In the search for these factors and substances, Professor Old also paid attention to the work of Dr. William B. Coley who, 100 years ago, accidentally discovered that cancer patients who suffered from one or more infections – such as those which can be caused by staphylococcal or streptococcal bacterial infections – survived longer or could even be described as having been 'cured'. The tumor shrank or was at least temporarily inhibited in its development.

Dr. Coley prepared a solution of so-called 'defused' streptococci and injected this solution, which acquired the name 'Coley's toxin', into cancer patients. Other physicians could not confirm his results. It was his daughter who, in an analysis of 896 successful cases, first demonstrated that there actually was something in Coley's toxin that worked against cancer. But what was it?

It appeared to be a mechanism that was stimulated by various bacteria. Such other substances as *Corynebacterium parvum* or the *BCG* vaccine obtained from a modified tubercle bacillus had already been employed as supportive therapy in the treatment measures for cancer and had led to positive reactions. This mechanism was clarified by Professor Old more than 20 years ago. Some bacteria even produce substances that stimulate the macrophages to liberate a factor which attacks cancer cells and destroys them.

This substance bears the scientific name *'tumor necrosis factor'* or TNF. Not only is it able to attack cancer cells selectively, it is also active against cells which have been infected by viruses.

Higher mammals have possessed this astonishing mechanism for millions of years. It has worked for millions of years in humans as well. When we suffer from an infection caused by bacteria, fungi or some viruses, one of the answers of the immune system is the release of this mediator substance TNF which attacks cancerous and virus-infected cells.

Unfortunately, we are now in the process of paralyzing this mechanism which is probably our best natural method of destroying the continually developing cancer cells and fighting the constant bombardment by viruses to which we are subjected. We do this by making use of the achievements of modern medicine prematurely, too frequently and to too great an extent when we immediately attack the slightest infection with antibiotics, cortisone and other infection-suppressant drugs.

If we immediately combat 'banal infections' or fevers up to 40 °C (104 °F) in this manner, we may paralyze our defenses against cancer and viral infections. Afterall, the fever is also a product of our body's defenses that is stimulated with the aid of TNF. We notice the activation of large quantities of TNF by such typical signs as tiredness and lassitude which are associated with infections and high fevers.

Our readiness to bear bodily discomfort is not very great. We wish to feel fit again as soon as possible and we therefore demand that our physicians prescribe the best possible drugs. It is generally believed that the best medicine is that which frees us most quickly from the symptoms of the disease. This seems to be an unintentional inducement on the part of the physician and patient to weaken the defense system and, among other things, to lose a magnificent chance of acting specifically against only the renegades which have developed from the body's own cells; against cancer cells and cells infected with viruses. When a patient suffers from cancer or viral disease, it is often said, "he has never been ill." Exactly, perhaps that is the problem, the patient has not suffered the protective infections which he or she normally would have had once or twice yearly.

The physician could now possibly tell the patient that he could prescribe a modern drug against cancer or viral disease, namely just that TNF which was previously suppressed. However, not the TNF the body produces and secretes for itself, but the TNF produced by genetic engineering.

Therapeutic tests, however, have so far been disappointing. TNF is particularly effective when the tumor mass is still small. TNF produced by genetic engineering has only been studied experimentally in substantially advanced cancers and there have frequently been severe side effects. Furthermore, the preparation is also quite expensive.

There are drugs that cause macrophages to release more TNF. One of these is a Japanese fungus extract, another is interferon, which is now produced by genetic engineering as well. These drugs can also produce severe side effects and pain. Their high price and limited positive results in experimental trials on cancer patients are factors which inhibit their general use, at least for the present.

This means that all those people who have any risk at all of suffering from cancer should do everything in their power to help their bodies to combat cancer cells and viruses in a natural manner. Since, as far as we know, our body only possesses a single weapon system for distinguishing between healthy and unhealthy cells, and destroying these unhealthy cells, the main objective must be to reinforce the immune system and to promote the release of TNF.

The recommendation of an increasing number of physicians is that 'banal' infections normally only involving a few days weakness on the part of the patient should be allowed to take their course under medical supervision and treatment with only supportive measures. It is best not to drop the temperature of every slight fever with antipyretics since this interferes with the battle of the immune system against the pathogen.

Our bodies are quite capable of producing and releasing small amounts of TNF without the stimulation of bacteria or some viruses. The secretion of TNF can also be stimulated by some vegetable components in the diet. The organism may then use the TNF which was set free to destroy individual cancer cells and cells infected by viruses.

However, the protection provided is only sufficient to keep in check what might be called the normal formation of cancer-like cells and the normal rate of viral infection in a body not exposed to excessive risk.

Nevertheless, such 'normality' is not very normal under the conditions of our civilization, rather it is the exception. Our life styles, diets, the environment and other circumstances lead to our almost automatic dependency on a greater than normal external stimulation of the immune system, particularly when elderly.

Ever more scientists recognize that there is probably no better principle for the protection from cancer and for combating cancer than keeping the body in an optimal condition to fulfill this task and to do that by means which are as natural as possible and which produce the fewest possible side effects. That is the reason why many millions of dollars are being spent at the moment in searching for such means and methods, and in discovering their basis, as well as ensuring their safety and applicability.

In the Austrian Cancer Research Institute at the University of Vienna, Dr. Lucia Desser has been studying the question of whether the success obtained in many cancer patients with the enzyme mixtures (oncologic and anti-inflammatory enzyme mixtures) could perhaps be the result of their stimulating the macrophages to release the tumor necrosis factor, TNF.

For this purpose, Dr. Desser treated cells with the enzyme mixtures and with the individual enzymes they contain. She also added the substance LPS (lipopolysaccharide) to the cells. LPS is the substance contained in the cell membranes of bacteria which brings about the formation and secretion of TNF. She found that the enzyme mixtures and the individual enzymes brought about a considerable secretion of TNF. According to her study, the enzyme mixtures proved to be of similar potency as the bacterial substances. LPS is now available as a commercial reagent. It is felt to be equivalent to the 'endotoxin' released from gram-negative bacteria which, when released in large amounts during certain infections, is known to be responsible for septic shock. LPS in small quantities is known to promote TNF induction, as well as macrophage activation and induction.

Since then, great efforts have been made to discover exactly what types of cancer respond best to the enzymatically stimulated TNF. The effect is not always the same, it differs for certain types of human and animal cancer. Then again, TNF stimulation, according to the enzyme scientists, requires a different enzyme dose depending on the cancer involved. They reported that some cancers die off completely and undergo necrosis after the administration of relatively low doses of the oncologic enzyme mixtures, for example, whereas other forms of cancer require much higher doses over a longer period of time.

The limits and possibilities

All this makes it sound as if enzyme therapy might be an alternative to the scalpel, radiation and chemotherapy for every case of cancer. This is certainly not the case, but according to the European physicians and research scientists, versatile enzyme therapy is acquiring a firm place in the prophylaxis, treatment and particularly in the follow-up care of carcinoma.

Afterall, according to them, enzyme therapy fulfills two criteria already set down by Paul Ehrlich, namely, that two factors must always be taken into consideration in cancer genesis and cancer growth; the defense power of the body and the malignancy of the growth. The researchers report that exactly these two factors must also be taken into account in enzyme therapy.

The European researchers are convinced that they "have demonstrated beyond all doubt that enzyme mixtures are capable of restoring the immune system by degrading the pathogenic immune complexes." In this context, they interpret this to mean, in particular, that the macrophages are reactivated and thereby aided in secreting the ideal armament, TNF.

Then again, they have reported that, "the enzyme mixtures are able to attack two dangerous properties of the cancer cells; they can degrade the fibrin, both unmasking the cancer cell antigens and thus removing the glue with which they attach themselves to vessel walls and tissues."

According to the scientists, this means that the more immune complex-degrading enzymes, and the more fibrinolytic enzymes which are present in the body, the greater is the chance that the defense system will be able to identify the individual cancer cells, unmask even their fibrin-coated enclaves, and make the fight against cancer cells even more effective by contributing to the breakdown of undegraded immune complexes. In this way, macrophages can be activated more effectively to transport them away.

The scientists also believe that this means people exposed to an increased risk of cancer can reduce this risk by taking the enzyme mixture directed against that particular cancer.

They also recommend the enzymes before and after cancer surgery "in order to compensate for the weakening of the immune system which always accompanies every surgical intervention."

Enzyme therapy for the treatment of cancer is also under investigation in hospitals. A significant number of oncologists in Germany, Italy and France already use enzymes for their cancer patients in the hospital. More recently, oncologists in the United States are starting to pay attention to this treatment and looking at the possibilities this presents.

The European enzymologists feel that almost all tumors accessible to injection needles can be treated by direct injection of enzyme mixtures into the tumor, to initiate its disintegration or, in certain cases, even cause its complete disintegration. Whenever surgery, radiation or chemotherapy is impossible or no longer sensible, the administration of enzyme mixtures by injection, microenema or tablet can at least achieve a mitigatory or palliative effect.

Furthermore, enzyme therapy has also been used as adjuvant therapy in combination with more traditional treatments. Scientists conducting recent radiotherapy studies in Europe concluded that when enzymes are administered concomitantly with radiation, somewhat lower radiation doses can be administered to produce the same effect. In addition, they also concluded that a higher dose of the enzyme mixture helps to protect from the feared radiation sickness and from some of the other adverse effects connected with radiation therapy. They claim that if the patient is provided with sufficient enzymes at the same time, the dosages used in the standard chemotherapy can also be reduced somewhat and the side effects of chemotherapy can be made less of a burden while still achieving the same effect.

They also pointed out that the appropriate administration of the enzyme mixture is often accompanied by an improvement in the morale of the cancer patients. Reportedly, the patients regain their appetite, put on weight, cease being depressed and feel considerably more alive, both physically and mentally.

Scientific articles have been published concerning the use of oral and systemic enzyme therapy for various forms of cancer which provide the interested physician with additional information. They cannot all be listed here, but some are included in the reference list for the benefit of interested readers or physicians.

Never forget the follow-up

Oncologists appear to agree on one very important recommendation that can make a significant difference regarding patients who have already been treated for cancer. Namely, that after strenuous chemotherapy or radiation therapy, the follow-up should always include optimal rules for avoiding any factors or activities which interfere with the patient's resistance to disease. This unfortunately does not always take place since the patient is frequently sent home with good wishes for the future, but is not provided with sufficient explanations concerning the best rules for the prevention of aggravating factors.

In particular, this applies to people who, as the physicians say, are 'free of macroscopic tumors', meaning those patients with no tumors visible in the various studies, including X-rays. It is well-known that up to 80% of these 'tumor-free' patients will eventually suffer recurrence of tumor growth. Although local recurrences may occur, this often occurs in the form of generalized nests of cancer cells, or metastases, which may spread regionally or to distant sites as well as throughout the entire body, rather than in the form of a solid tumor. Afterall, most cancer patients do not ultimately die as a result of the primary tumor, but instead due to such multiple involvement of the entire body.

Previously, low doses of certain chemotherapeutic agents were prescribed in such cases for long-term therapy. An attempt was made to preventively kill all newly formed cells in the body as they divided. Purely statistically, this may have had the effect of reducing the chance of new cancer cell formation, but there is no doubt that it also had the effect of further weakening the defense system as well. Today, there are scarcely any oncologists who are of the opinion that long-term treatment with drugs to inhibit cell division can lead to worthwhile results in cancer patients free of macroscopic tumors.

Instead, ever more physicians have recognized that other measures to help strengthen the whole body are more appropriate.

Prevention starts with avoidance of undue emotional stress and making space for proper relaxation and recreation. Avoidance of exposure to pollutants, such as smoking, smog, toxins, environmental carcinogens, excessive ultraviolet light, excessive alcohol or substance abuse become most important. Emphasis has also been placed on an immediate change in diet, recommending a high proportion of fresh salads, vegetables, and other raw wholefoods, such as fresh fruit, grains and nuts, while avoiding highly refined, overcooked or high sugar foods. The inclusion of multiple vitamins, supplemented with vitamins A, E and C, and especially of such trace elements as zinc, copper, selenium and germanium, has also been recommended.

According to the European scientists, enzyme therapy has earned a special position as an ethical, rational and highly promising preventive measure. It certainly makes sense to prevent the formation of cancer cells. However, since this is not always possible, at least the goal should be to combat the new cancer cells being formed continually, when they are still at the stage of being either single cells, or small metastases containing small numbers of cells searching for an anchoring place in the blood or lymph vessels. The European scientists feel that prophylaxis for metastatic spread should definitely include the use of enzymes.

The European regimen for prevention is of interest. They emphasize that it is not necessary to swallow numerous enzyme tablets continuously for this purpose. As a rule of thumb, only one oncologic enzyme mixture tablet is taken daily for a week, followed by a pause of three weeks. This schedule is then repeated. They feel that, "the large dose of enzymes contained in one tablet will have a specific anticancer effect on those metastases which have taken about four weeks to develop. If the body is also provided with assistance in strengthening the defenses by means of a healthier way of life as previously mentioned, patients will have a better chance of keeping the illness under control. This applies to that patient who has been discharged from the hospital after treat-

ment for cancer, or even to any persons who might have a certain
risk of suffering from cancer."

When the breast is in danger

We should also briefly discuss a persistent and difficult disorder
associated with the treatment of breast cancer. This disorder is
called lymphedema and represents a form of rather exaggerated
swelling. Some women who have been operated on for removal of
the breast and subsequently had radiation therapy of the armpit
suffer from lymphedema of the arm. This swelling can sometimes
reach massive proportions. This can have a considerable impact
on the quality of the woman's life and also reduces the general
prospects of healing. The European scientists report that they
have been able to prevent the development of lymphedema by the
simple prophylactic administration of the anti-inflammatory
enzyme mixtures twice daily for two years, starting immediately
after surgery or radiation therapy. Since breast cancer at the time
of diagnosis has more recently been recognized as a systemic disease, there has been a substantial decrease in the use of the more
radical surgery that is more likely to result in lymphedema. Nevertheless, anyone who has experienced the suffering that such a
lymphedema can cause will realize how important its long-term
prevention can be.

Another important application of oral enzyme therapy was
reported by investigators from the Janker Radiation Clinic in
Bonn. Many women, especially younger women, have a fear of
breast cancer when they suddenly feel a lump in their breast. It is
estimated that over 16 million women in the United States and
Germany have discovered such lumps and fear that they will have
to undergo surgery, lose their breast or even die of cancer.

However, lumps and painful inflammatory changes in the
breast are no sure sign that a malignant process is taking place.
Tissue samples are often taken or operations performed which

demonstrate that the growth is benign. This is often called 'fibro-cystic disease of the breast' (mastopathia cystica benigna).

Reports from studies conducted at the Janker Clinic in Germany have indicated that these benign lumps, in their experience, improve considerably and in some cases even disappear within a few weeks after the administration of polyenzyme mixtures twice daily plus 1,000 mg vitamin E. In this manner, the Janker Clinic reported 90% success in controlling these benign lumps and other painful inflammatory processes of the breast. They indicated that, should the complaints reappear later, a further course of enzyme therapy and vitamin E usually brings about the same results. They describe the treatment as "an almost harmless sounding recipe, but one which is certainly capable of freeing many women from anxiety and sparing them other unpleasant coursesof treatment." Of course, lesions that persist for several weeks need to be evaluated by physicians experienced in the diagnosis of breast tumors, and mammography and/or biopsy may be required.

Finally, mention must be made of other diseases that frequently attack cancer patients. When the host defenses are diminished, some enemies can therefore take hold. One such example is shingles, medically known as herpes zoster. This represents an attack by a virus. Like thrombosis, it often occurs in cancer patients. More information about enzyme treatment of shingles can be found in the next chapter.

Chapter 16

Viruses: Dead or alive?

Dead or alive? No one knows exactly. You might say that viruses are dead because they do not metabolize and cannot multiply of their own accord. You could also say they are alive because they can penetrate foreign cells, present foreign cells with the plans for making more viruses like themselves and persuade these cells to turn out faithful copies of this invading virus. Most people think of them as alive.

Whatever they are, these beings are so incredibly tiny that they can only be seen with the aid of an extremely powerful electron microscope. They are nevertheless among the most dangerous enemies to our health. We scarcely know how to attack them, how to slow them down or how to get rid of them.

Suspicion fell on them whenever the origin of a disease puzzled us. It has also been suggested that cancer is caused by viruses. This theory has had militant defenders and vigorous opponents, and both were right; cancer is not a 'viral disease' in general, but some viruses have been shown to cause some types of cancer.

Such viruses are known as cancer viruses. The American cancer researchers Baltimore, Dulbecco and Temin received the 1975 Nobel prize for medicine because they were able to demonstrate the interaction of cancer viruses and the genetic material in the cells of the body. The cancer viruses slip into normal cells and change them so that they become cancer cells, i.e. enemies of the body (Figure 42).

One class of viruses which has been incriminated in this business of transforming a normal cell into a cancer cell is the herpes family of viruses. They comprise a family of viruses with different structures and different effects on the organism they infect, but they are all related to each other and possess similar characteristics.

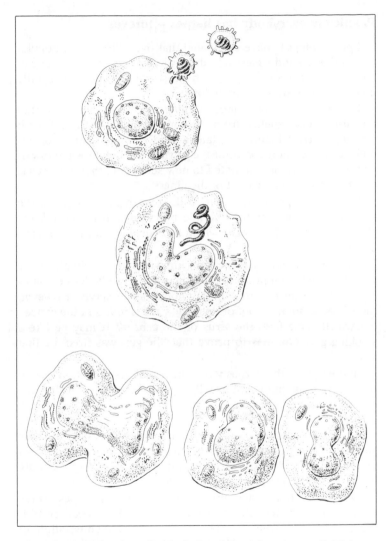

Figure 42: Viruses invade a cell of the body and alter it in such a way that it degenerates to produce replicating cancer cells

Practically everybody has herpes – forever

Epidemiologists have calculated that over 90% of the population of Europe and America is already infected with at least one of the six basic forms of herpes, with viruses which, and there is little doubt, are present in the body forever.

In other words, the diabolical thing about these viruses is that the virus is not expelled from the body after the first infection, it remains there, it hibernates, latent, hidden in some niche of our body. Under certain conditions, e.g. when the defenses are low, it awakes again and is stimulated to new activity, so that the virus is able to bring on a new bout of the illness.

It has been postulated that, with some types of viruses, the reaction of the body to the first infection causes this virus to bring about dramatic cell changes which subsequently can lead to cancer cells.

Thus, it is thought that the virus known as herpes simplex virus type 2 is a potential producer of cancer and must be looked on as one of the suspect causes of carcinoma of the cervix. However, there is no absolute proof of this. The virus is found in the cancer, but which came first, the virus or the cancer? It may be like a smoking gun. One has to prove that 'the gun was fired' by that virus.

In the case of the herpes virus, the actual first infection resembles a severe flu, but is not usually regarded as being a lasting disorder by either the patient or the physician. One should emphasize that it is simply not the case that every attack on our normal body cells by herpes virus automatically results in some sort of cancer. In fact, at present, the papovavirus which causes venereal warts, also known as Condylomas, is felt to be more closely associated with cancer of the cervix.

Other conditions have also been attributed to herpes. These include, for instance, stomach ulcers, which have been considered, but not proven, to merely represent a manifestation of renewed herpes attacks. More recently, other infectious agents, including a germ called Hemophylus pylorus, have also been incriminated as the cause of stomach ulcers and antibiotic treatments have been proposed.

The virus of the herpes group which causes *shingles* occupies a special position. The disease is known as zoster and the virus is known as the varicella-zoster virus. The first infection by this virus does not actually result in shingles. The disease that develops is ordinary chicken pox.

When the chicken pox resulting from this primary infection has subsided, we might think that the virus has been killed off and driven from the body, but this is not quite true. Numerous zoster viruses remain behind in the body as if asleep. They take permanent residence in a swelling of the nerve known as the dorsal ganglion and stay there like a prisoner in a jail until our defenses falter and the prisoner escapes.

Attacking when our defenses are down

The viruses awaken when our bodies are weakened. At this time they travel along the nerve unto the surface skin and have a good chance of penetrating our healthy cells, forcing them to make copies of the invaders in order to be able to continue their attack. By attacking the nerves and skin cells, they produce painful blisters. This reactivation, usually decades after the first attack, is known as shingles. Shingles thus occurs when our bodies are weakened by a severe disease, such as cancer, by other infections or by drugs which suppress the defense system. In addition, some scientists feel that such mental stresses as mourning, depression or the oft-cited stress of everyday life also play a role in the virus reactivation causing shingles.

Suddenly, there they are, hordes of them! Simultaneously awakened and activated, the zoster viruses begin to attack our cells. As a result of the primary infection with chicken pox, our bodies have now produced a whole range of specific antibodies against these viruses. Indeed, these antibodies helped to cure the chicken pox. Some of these specialists, the antibodies, are still in the ranks of our defenders.

As soon as the zoster viruses awaken from their hibernation, the alarm is sounded by these specific antibodies which multiply rapidly and attack the foreign characteristics of the zoster viruses, the antigens.

It is not only necessary to arrest all viruses; each complete virus is accompanied by multiple incomplete virus particles with pieces that can also penetrate our cells. They may not force the host cell to fabricate complete viruses, but they alter the host cell to such an extent that it is no longer recognized as being part of the body and is therefore treated as an enemy.

We now know what happens when enemy particles amass, especially in a body whose defenses are weakened, and where excess antibodies have formed immune complexes. Unfortunately, these immune complexes are only partially degraded on account of the weakness of the immune system. All those immunological responses typical of immune complex diseases occur, as discussed in previous chapters.

Shingles or herpes zoster is just such a disease. The undegraded immune complexes formed from zoster antigens and antibodies have a tendency to lodge on what are known as receptors of the nerve cells. The structure of these cells has already been altered by the virus. The immune complexes adhering to the length of the nerve activate enzymes triggering the complement cascade intended for the lysis of bacteria or viruses. This again causes inflammation, damage to the nerve cells, pain (at times excruciating), and the typical symptoms of shingles; small blisters of the skin, swollen lymph nodes, itching, burning, irritation and a general feeling of fatigue.

Until a few years ago, scientific texts on the treatment of shingles were pretty much in agreement, it was not possible to effectively treat the causes of this disease. The blisters were covered with creams and ointments, including cortisone, and vitamin B_{12}, gamma globulin, lysine or numerous other medications were prescribed. However, physicians were of the opinion that these were of little or no help and that, just as with a common cold, the only thing to do was to control the pain and wait for shingles to heal by itself. In two or three weeks, the zoster is normally healed and can be forgotten unless *post-herpetic neuralgia* occurs. This is a form of extreme sensitivity and very severe recurrent pains, usually triggered by a light touch of the affected skin such as by clothing or bed covers, by the shower or wind, or at times spontaneously. The neuralgia is a frequent sequel of shingles, particularly among the elderly. The excruciating nerve pains can last for months or even years, and rarely even for a lifetime. The neuralgia is virtually resistant to medical treatment. Scientists have postulated that the neuralgia is due to immune complexes triggering complement and other changes which damage the nerve.

Many physicians are limited in the treatment of shingles and particularly in that of post-herpetic neuralgia. In recent years, the drug acyclovir has offered help for the shingles, but not for the neuralgia.

European experience advocates the use of oral enzyme mixtures in the treatment of shingles and in the prevention of post-herpetic neuralgia. The enzymes, according to them, act specifically against immune complexes. Traditional physicians will question the rationale of the administration of oral enzymes in the treatment of a virus until they learn about the role of immune complexes.

Papilloma viruses and plant viruses:
From dairy cow to orchid

It was Professor Max Wolf who came upon this therapeutic approach when he visited a dairy farm in South Florida after the Second World War and treated dairy cattle suffering from papillomatosis, benign tumors on the skin ranging up to the size of a fist. The cause and appearance of these lesions is similar to the previously mentioned human papovavirus producing the condylomata acuminatae. In those days, the enzyme mixtures he used were not so refined as those we now apply. He injected it into the hides of the cattle in the vicinity of the tumors. The tumors fell off after a few days, the cattle were restored to health.

Since Max Wolf was aware that papillomatosis was caused by a virus, he concluded that the enzymes had deactivated the viruses. He speculated that the enzymes had degraded the proteinaceous envelope or 'foot' of the virus which the virus uses to attach itself to normal cells. According to Dr. Wolf, the enzyme treatment thereby made it impossible for the virus to penctrate the wall of the host cell.

Wolf then applied the enzymes to virus-infected plants as well. He applied tobacco mosaic virus to bean plants and found that all plants not previously treated with the enzyme mixture had become infected. However, if the bean plants were previously treated with enzyme mixtures, they withstood inoculation with virus without damage and only exhibited a mild reaction.

Reportedly, similar results were obtained in an experiment involving valuable orchids which were severely infected by a virus at a nursery. They were treated with enzymes and could eventually be freed from the disease.

Horticulturalists have not as yet adopted this method, but more and more veterinarians have realized that they can use this enzyme therapy as a simple method of treatment for some animal diseases which previously posed difficulties. They were less interested in why and how the treatment worked than in the fact that it did work.

Thus, they used such enzyme mixtures for the treatment of bovine papillomatosis and bovine pneumonia which is particularly prevalent in Lower Bavaria in late winter and can take the lives of thousands of cattle. Veterinarians then came upon the idea of testing the enzyme mixtures on virally-induced equine distemper which is greatly feared among owners of valuable race horses. They concluded that the treatment also proved to be successful.

A report from Chad in Africa that a camel pox epidemic was threatening economic catastrophe led Dr. Dunkel to visit the country and arrange for the camels to be treated with the potent enzyme mixture. The viral infection which bears a close resemblance to human smallpox was rapidly brought under control. While in Chad, Dr. Dunkel also investigated the effect of the enzymes on viral leukemia in chickens. He reported that chicken viral leukemia could be adequately treated in this manner, but that it cost more than the poultry were worth.

These veterinary successes gave some human physicians the courage to test enzyme therapy for the treatment of viral diseases in man.

Protection from severe nerve pain

In 1964, Dr. Dorrer of the Prien Hospital on the banks of the Chiemsee first administered the oncologic enzyme mixtures to 24 patients with shingles. The results on which he reported were impressive! According to him, when the enzyme treatment was started on a high dosage scale within 24 hours of the first appearance of the blisters, the pain ceased within three days and the blisters formed scabs much quicker than is normally the case. The most important result reported by Dr. Dorrer, however, was that not one single patient later suffered from the dreaded post-herpetic neuralgia, the pains of which can be so severe that some patients have even been driven to suicide.

The publication of Dr. Dorrer's results was the signal for other physicians to follow his example. Dr. Bartsch, head physician of the Wald Sanitarium, an outpatient cancer clinic with 200 beds, in Urbachtal, Germany, is probably one of the foremost physicians in this field.

According to him, the treatment of zoster was a problem of particular urgency since a relationship between 'cancer and

zoster' has been acknowledged in medicine, similar to the relationship between 'cancer and thrombosis'. For this reason, he
began with a comparative study where a group of cancer patients
suffering from shingles were treated with large doses of enzyme
mixtures in 1968. Here, a second group was treated with the drugs
usually prescribed for herpes zoster.

Dr. Bartsch abandoned the investigation for ethical reasons
after he had treated a total of 23 patients. He simply was no
longer willing to treat patients with the usual methods since, in his
opinion, the superiority of the enzyme preparation had already
become clearly evident.

Since then, several hundred herpes zoster patients have been
treated in this hospital. The subsequent publications of Dr.
Bartsch reconfirmed the initial reports of success, "At this time,
we regard the treatment of herpes zoster with proteolytic enzymes
as being the therapy which is most effective, free from side effects
and most optimal", he wrote.

There was, however, one reservation. He had noted that,
"longer periods of illness and of pain for the patient are usually
the result of delaying the start of therapy." According to Dr. Bartsch and other researchers, it is scarcely possible to exert a favorable effect on the chronic pain of post-herpetic neuralgia if
enzyme therapy is commenced too late, like weeks after the start
of the disorder. If treatment is started at an earlier point in time
and the doses are adequate, it is possible to speak of successful
prophylaxis against post-herpetic neuralgia in their opinion.

More recent studies by Dr. Michael Kleine have confirmed the
previous reports. In addition, in a double blind, cross-over study,
Dr. Kleine compared the oral enzyme mixtures with oral acyclovir
in the treatment of zoster and reported that both drugs were
equally effective in reducing the severity, morbidity and duration
of the illness. However, according to his report, the enzymes were
able to prevent the post-herpetic neuralgia while the acyclovir did
not. Furthermore, the enzyme treatment was found to be less
expensive.

This enzymatic method of treating viral infections, primarily by eliminating the nondegraded and thereby pathogenic immune complexes, has recently been under discussion for the treatment of what has until now been the most problematical of all viral diseases, AIDS.

Zoster and AIDS, the same principle?

There actually are certain parallels between herpes zoster and AIDS. AIDS also begins with a seemingly-harmless, initial infection with HIV virus and only later is there a second, serious attack. A person just infected with AIDS after the first exposure merely suffers a flu-like illness with slight fever and a general feeling of fatigue. Many assume it is only an unimportant flu and soon forget it because it normally disappears quite quickly. This first phase corresponds with the chicken pox of patients infected with zoster.

Analogous with other viral infections, the body of a person infected with AIDS produces specific antibodies. These specific antibodies directed against HIV AIDS virus can be detected in the blood and are important for diagnosis. If these antibodies are present, the person is 'HIV positive', although this does not mean that he or she is already suffering from AIDS.

Afterall, it can be many years before the inactive HIV viruses present in the body are activated by additional stress or when the immune system begins to falter, thus setting in motion the disease process that deteriorates in stages. After an indefinite length of time, the HIV positive person may develop generalized swelling of lymph nodes (the lymphadenopathy syndrome) and the patients subsequently develop multiple medical problems (ARC or AIDS related complex). Eventually, the condition leads to full-blown AIDS with immune system collapse and usually ends in death. The precipitant for the progression, for instance, can be an infection, or the administration of immunosuppressive drugs which further depress the body's own defenses.

Immunosuppressive antiviral drugs are capable of inhibiting viral proliferation. However, the price which must be paid for this reduced viral proliferation is very high since the suppressed defenses make the body helpless against other infections. For this reason, such drugs are generally prescribed only in cases where the immune system is already weakened completely, so that no further weakening is possible. Thus, they probably should only be used as a last resort to treat the advanced stages of AIDS where they may slow down the further development of the disease to some extent. Another problem with the immunosuppressive, antiviral treatments is their severe side effects. It becomes obvious that AIDS, to date, cannot be brought to a halt with immunosuppressive, anitviral drugs and that death may in fact be hastened.

Anyone who considers the degree to which the fate of an HIV positive patient is dependent on the strength of the immune system will have second thoughts about the use of immunosuppressive drugs. Most physicians will not even think of using these defense-weakening drugs in the intermediate stages of the HIV disorder, particularly before the complete array of AIDS symptoms has broken out, since whatever immunity is left needs to be preserved to the outmost.

Scientists familiar with the immunity of illnesses advocate the notion that viral infections should be combated with treatment reinforcing the body's defenses. They reason that the body must marshal all the surveillance and defense methods available to it in order to oppose the disease with some degree of success.

Many factors need to be considered in preserving the body's defenses. Avoidance of exposures to the previously mentioned conditions known to weaken our immune system is paramount. Likewise, relieving the body of environmental and metabolic toxins by a sensible life style, healthy exercise and proper diet becomes most important in the HIV illness.

The use of many biological response modifiers and similar methods aimed at strengthening the body is under continued investigation and appears promising. The entire concept of prevention needs to be considered and adapted to each patient, and then followed strictly.

Just don't weaken

Apart from this general assistance which strengthens the defenses and thus delays the onset of clinical AIDS, providing direct and specific assistance is naturally mandatory as well.

Scientists think that one of the aims must be to stimulate the helper cells of the immune system which have been inhibited by the HIV virus. It is even more important to activate the macrophages from their virus-dependent inhibition. The inhibition of the macrophages which renders them unable to perform their usual function of viral destruction is felt by many scientists to be the result of the immune complexes formed by the AIDS viruses and the antibodies of the immune system.

They feel that the overabundance of these inhibitory immune complexes is one of the principal factors that makes AIDS so dangerous. The immune complexes locked to the viral antigens are not degraded because the AIDS virus attacks and paralyzes the defense cells necessary for this purpose. In addition, the HIV antigens locked in the immune complexes react with the helper cells and bind themselves to them. The complement system, alarmed by this abortive 'immune complex-helper cell-HIV virus tangle' destroys the helper cells coupled to the HIV viruses because it recognizes them as being enemies due to the fact that they are attached to the virus containing tangle.

Ever more scientists confirm that the destruction of helper cells is a primary reason for the fatal consequences of the 'acquired immune deficiency syndrome', and this is felt to be caused by the complement attack on the immune complexes.

For these reasons, the European scientists propose enzyme therapy in order to promote mobilization of the immune complexes in the tissues, bringing them into the circulation and available for further endogenous and/or therapeutic enzymatic degradation. They view this as a logical, effective and safe medical assistance in the treatment of AIDS. Several hospitals in America, Germany and France, as well as numerous physicians in private practice, are currently applying this principle in the treatment of AIDS patients. In the United States, this treatment is the subject of a research investigation at a major medical center.

Once again, the European scientists have postulated that the administration of enzyme mixtures, particularly that of the anti-inflammatory combinations, is able to release tissue-bound immune complexes into the circulation and expose them to further enzymatic degradation. "When this is accomplished, the inhibition of the macrophage activity is ended and the erroneous destruction of the necessary immune system helper cells by complement is prevented."

They feel that the immune deficiency is thus reduced and that further advance of the AIDS symptoms is slowed down significantly. They report that the patient remains HIV positive but can remain symptom-free much longer. However, it is still just as impossible to remove all HIV viruses from the body as it is to eliminate other viruses which have gained access to the organism completely, and the patient will remain HIV positive. Medicine is searching for a specific cure, but none has thus far been found.

Some of this systemic enzyme therapy work is documented in clinical studies that have been under way since 1985. In some of the studies, the treatment of these patients was not limited to enzyme therapy. The therapists also administered other biological response modifiers together with therapies known to augment the defenses, as well as vitamin A.

According to the scientists, these measures produced an appreciable improvement in the symptoms, particularly in patients in the earlier stages of the disease – LAS (lymphadenopathy syndrome) and ARC (AIDS related complex). The reported improvement was particularly true for neurological disorders, the ability to concentrate, depression and also for inflammation of the lungs, coughing, respiratory distress, general debility, loss of appetite, loss of weight, diarrhea, visual disturbances, fever and walking impediments.

In the various studies utilizing enzyme therapy for HIV disease reported so far, the researchers have concluded that the improvement of the general condition was also reflected in improvement of such blood parameters as the lymphocyte (T-helper-cells) and erythrocyte counts, the erythrocyte sedimentation rate and other tests. They reported that the numbers of these cells increased under this therapy only in those patients who prior to the start of therapy did not suffer too great a deficiency of helper cells.

The Medical Enzyme Research Institute published the following conclusions regarding the results of the controlled clinical studies so far completed:

1. Progression of the early stages of HIV disease is significantly limited by the enzyme treatment. The patients' symptoms are appreciably improved.

2. In the case of people who are HIV positive, enzyme treatment can delay the onset of disease symptoms. In some cases, this delay appears to continue indefinitely, symptomatically representing a substantial improvement.

3. A low-grade helper-cell suppression can be improved by enzyme therapy.

4. The occurrence of infectious disease, and possibly of malignant disease, have become less common than in the control groups. This was felt to be due to increased macrophage activity, the reinstated degradation of foreign cells and improvements in the helper-cells' defense mechanisms.

All this makes it sound as if there is nothing in this life that cannot be improved, reinforced or healed by the administration of enzymes. According to the European scientists, there is some truth in that. They feel that enzymes provide not only a healthy life, but a long one as well. They also feel that enzymes even come to our aid in the process which is not spared by any of us, the process of aging.

Chapter 17

Age: The best brake

Everyone wants to live to a ripe old age, but nobody wants to be old. All of us are concerned with the thought of growing old and dying one day. Some people are filled with dismay and others give up completely, their fear of death prevents them from enjoying life to the fullest. Most people would like to delay the aging process and push their deaths into the distant future.

We all secretly hope that during our lifetime someone will come and say, "Eureka! We know the mechanism of death and we can stop it. We have conquered death. Anyone who wants to, can have unlimited life."

Let us now ignore the question of whether unlimited life is worth striving for, whether it might not herald the end of human society. Let us rather turn to the 'mechanism' which ensures that every living thing eventually dies. We are on the trail of such a mechanism, and scientists now know that not all living organisms die.

There is such a thing as quasi-eternal life. In our own bodies as well. Our bodies always house a few or even many cancer cells and they are primitive things which do not contain the inborn mortality mechanism. Given the right conditions, they could theoretically live for ever.

In the laboratory, several organisms that are long-living and can multiply themselves indefinitely are used for cell culture. For instance, a particularly vigorous line of cervical cancer cells has been crossed with macrophages to yield a hybrid line known as 'HeLa U 927'. These can be considered to be quasi-immortal macrophages. Certain tissues or organs, such as a chick's heart, can be kept alive for indefinite lengths of time in certain cell suspensions.

However, every cell normally stops metabolizing and dies after a certain length of time. It is normally assumed that most of the cells of the human body are no longer capable of producing error-free copies after they have divided 45 or 50 times. The weakened cells that are now a source of danger to the body notice that for themselves. They decide on their own deaths, thus sacrificing themselves in the end for the good of the body as a whole. They 'commit suicide' by inserting particular receptors through their membranes. These are landing places for specific antibodies, or more effectively immune complexes, which then trigger the complement cascade of enzymes which ends in the enzymatic disintegration of the age-weakened cell.

This voluntary suicide of age-weakened cells is a decisively important mechanism in the process of 'cell molting', the process of cell renewal which takes place during every second of our lives, the replacement of aging cells by vigorous, new, perfectly-functioning cells.

Scientists ask the same questions concerning the life and death of a single cell that they do about the life and death of a person, "Does life terminate as a result of an accumulation of errors or is there a genetically incorporated mechanism triggered by a pre-chosen signal?"

The unfortunate people who suffer from neonatal progeria (Hutchinson-Gilford syndrome) or the Werner syndrome provide tragic evidence that the process of aging is controlled genetically. These syndromes involve the premature senility of children or young people either shortly after birth (*progeria*), or after the start of puberty (Werner syndrome). A genetic code that has run out of control turns such patients into senile old people within a few years so that they rapidly die of the typical diseases of old age. Another genetic condition, *acrogeria* or Gottron's syndrome, causes the aging to occur only on the distal extremities. Their general health and life expectancy are otherwise normal.

Death awaits in a chromosome

So, the signal for aging and death lies hidden in the genetic code. But where? In order to answer this question, Japanese and

American scientists have crossed human connective tissue cells with 'immortal' hamster cancer cells and investigated the hybrid cells obtained for changes in the genetic code which enables the hybrid cells to continue dividing endlessly, thereby endowing them with immortality. They discovered that a human gene which controls our aging processes is found in the first of our 23 chromosomes.

Theoretically, there is a possibility that genetic engineering could be used in the future to alter the set of human chromosomes and thereby delay aging. Similar processes have already been carried out, bringing about considerable increases in the life-spans of molds, worms, flies and mice. They pass on this greater life expectancy to further generations as well.

It is not yet possible to carry out such manipulations on the hereditary material of human beings. Our best chance is to be descendants from parents whose ancestors were particularly long-lived. This means that we possess a particular guarantee that chromosome 1 possesses an aging gene which comes into action late.

Naturally, this is not a guarantee against death, it is not even a guarantee of long life. A second factor responsible for the aging process which always has to be taken into account is the factor of ever increasing errors in the overall metabolic selectivity.

Although we cannot do much about some errors, for instance metabolic abnormalities as a result of genetically determined enzyme deficiencies, research is making great advances in this area and clinical trials of genetic replacement have already begun, for some diseases, as noted in the introduction. However, we can fortunately avoid most of the environmental and abuse errors that weaken the body and make it age prematurely. If we desire a longer and healthier life, we should take hold of this opportunity with both hands.

Eat little, live long

One possibility of giving the body an opportunity to survive longer lies in eating less. Numerous investigations have confirmed time and again what everyone could see in Germany during and after the War, a severely limited diet, particularly less meat and fat, does actually lead to a healthier and longer life. The fact that the statistical life expectancy has increased continually over the last decades is not a result of our behavior, but rather, thanks to medical advances, and particularly to a decrease in the infant death rate.

Anyone who inquires closely into the influence of food on life expectancy is most likely to realize the truth of the situation. Thus, Dr. Roy Walford, an immunologist at UCLA in Los Angeles, California, has succeeded in increasing the normal life-span of laboratory mice two or threefold by selecting the best, so-called 'major histocompatibility complex' for their genetic makeup. Since Dr. Walford has seen what tremendous damage a rich diet can cause to the immune system in his own studies, he does not rely on genetics to increase his own life-span, but instead has reduced his caloric intake by almost half. Again, in the laboratories of the National Toxicology Laboratory in Little Rock, Arkansas, there are thousands of rats and mice that live twice as long as normal because their diets have been reduced by 40%. Reportedly, the director of this laboratory and his assistants have also adjusted their menus in response to this example.

Naturally, we do not only eat too much, we also eat incorrectly, too quickly, too hot, too cold. We make all the mistakes that we have already talked about in the chapter on digestion. We perform too little exercise and we damage our health with smoking and other poisons, we expose ourselves to man-made pollutants (Figure 43).

If instead we were to live as reason and not pleasure tells us, we should, we would, come close to the ideal of living a healthy life to an advanced age. It has been estimated that a considerable adjustment in our way of life and a reduction of atmospheric and other pollution would reduce the number of chronic respiratory diseases by two thirds to three quarters.

Our unnatural way of life and man-made pollution cause disturbances to the human body, for example the large-scale production of so-called 'free radicals'. These are chaotically reacting molecules present in our bodies which contribute to many diseases from cancer to heart attacks and which are thought to be responsible for many premature aging processes.

Free radicals can also cause genetic damage when they react with our DNA. We won't get into that. The damage to proteins makes the point. Free radicals oxidize our cells so that they practically rust and normal metabolism is impossible for them. If the destructive rage of the free radicals is not stopped, they can weaken the whole body until illness and premature death results. There are researchers of old age (gerontologists) who believe that free radicals are the most important cause of the pathological aging processes.

Free radicals also play a discreditable role in the formation of cross linkages. Cross linkages are special bonds connecting amino acid chains. The cross linkages we are talking about are the undesired ones between protein chains which can occur in connective tissues and indeed in other tissues. The most evident damage this causes is to reduce the elasticity of the connective tissue. This is most easily tested by raising the skin on the back of the hand between two fingers and then releasing it.

If the fold of skin immediately becomes flat again, it has not yet been damaged and aged by cross linking (Figure 43). Crows feet of the eyes and wrinkles on the forehead are visible signs of connective tissue cross linking.

The connective tissue is made up of giant protein chains, some of which are arranged in spirals and some parallel to each other, which provide the tensile, extensive, flexile and compressive strengths of the connective tissue. Just like the springs and wires of a mattress or trampoline, they provide both elasticity and strength.

The ability of the protein chains to move depends on their being connected together without restricting one another. Think of the strings of a harp, they are firmly anchored and can nevertheless each vibrate elastically and return to the original tension when the vibration has stopped. However, if two adjacent harp strings were to be connected together they would no longer be able to vibrate so freely and would lose their elasticity.

The more errors our body makes as we age, the more cross linkages are produced. The less able the body is to cleave these cross linkages on account of lacking enzyme activity, the stiffer and more rigid, and lacking in functionality will be our connective tissue. Most important is to realize that tendons, muscles, nerve fibers, blood vessels and virtually most tissues are also damaged similarly (Figure 43).

To a certain extent, we can protect ourselves from the damage caused by free radicals by avoiding every influence that promotes their formation. The list is long and includes some things which most people like doing very much and do not care to do without. These people are therefore willing to accept the possibility of premature aging and perhaps premature death.

The influences that promote the formation of free radicals and cross linkages include prolonged and unprotected exposure to sunlight, certain types of UV radiation and radioactive radiation, nicotine, saturated fats and fats which have been overheated or exposed to the heat of a grill, industrial and other exhaust gases, and numerous other toxins and pollutants that we inhale, drink or eat and which are administered to us (Figure 44).

It is better to eat raw, non-toxic vegetables and fruits, a few carrots, some sweet peppers, apples, etc. every day. Fats should be consumed in the form of unsaturated vegetable oils or fish oils.

The disastrous effects of free radicals can also be limited by means of what are known as radical binders, as with 'rust preventives'. These are such antioxidants as vitamins E and C, the trace

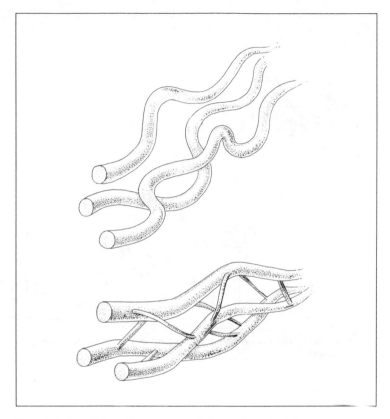

Figure 43: Cross linkage: Erroneous cross linkages of protein chains

element selenium which is active at the lowest dose levels, or such enzymatic radical binders as superoxide dismutase (SOD) and other hydrolytic enzymes. SOD, unfortunately, is inactivated in the gut and oral administration therefore appears to be ineffective.

According to the European scientists, the breakdown and inhibition of the formation of cross-linked protein chains is also car-

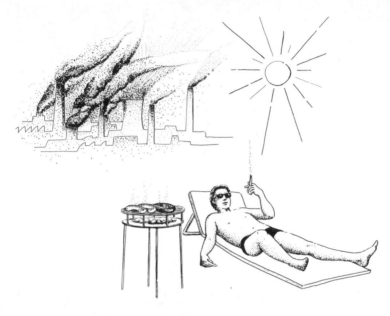

Figure 44: Factors which promote the development of free radicals and cross link-
           ages

ried out by the proteolytic enzymes present in the most frequently used enzyme mixtures. They postulate that when taken over long periods, they contribute in old age to the maintenance of elasticity of the tissue and hence to its improved function. They further remark that, "it is naturally impossible to slow down every form of aging. The provision of enzymes does not absolve us from the obligation to do everything to avoid as many metabolic errors as possible in order to prevent premature aging."

Just don't make mistakes

The percentage of senior citizens is constantly increasing. Strangely enough, few scientists devote themselves to the study of the aging process. A process that most people suffer eventually and which is certainly fatal in outcome. However, many gerontologists agree that there are only two routes to the long-term maintenance of health and prolongation of life; one is interference with the genetic code and the other is the reduction of the error rate in people's metabolism.

No organism operates completely without errors. Every instant, even at this very moment, there are about a billion cells in your body undergoing transformation, dividing, dying, being renewed. About 230,000 cells are created every second, that is about 20 billion per day. Every single cell transformation requires millions of quite specific biochemical steps which can only be carried out in the presence of exactly shaped enzymes and have to be carried out at a speed that can hardly be measured.

Naturally, errors are made. When the body is young and healthy, the immune system performs reliable corrections. However, these errors can occur throughout the entire body, meaning such errors can also occur in the immune system, that system whose duty it is to eradicate errors. This means that as the years go by, exactly the very same system intended to eradicate errors, to carry out repairs and to maintain health, becomes itself subject to errors. Errors in this region can have particularly serious consequences.

We ought to live our lives as natural, as healthy, as relaxed as possible, with sufficient exercise, with a natural and fresh diet, avoiding environmental and other poisons. Live this way – as our common sense tells us to, as we always intended to – and as the majority of people do not. This would be the simplest, cheapest and most effective brake on aging.

Otherwise, all that remains is a repair service for the damaged body. This repair service takes particular care of two forms of damage that generally occur with age, that caused by circulatory problems and that resulting from weaknesses of the immune system. In advanced countries, it is primarily cardiovascular diseases and cancer that cause the death of four out of five people. However, the chronic diseases that can make the lives of the elderly such a misery must also be considered, since the quality of life can be severely affected and, for some, this can be a 'living death'.

The blood supply problems of old age are the result of the ever decreasing activation of plasmin. Its decrease prevents adequate blood liquefaction, the formation of fibrin gains the upper hand. Blood clots then form which cause the blockage of the blood vessels and arteriosclerosis results. Calcification of the vessels also occurs. It all happens as described in the chapter on blood vessels. The reader is invited to read this chapter again.

According to the scientists, what has been said about the help provided for arteries and veins by enzymes naturally applies fully for the elderly who demonstrate more circulatory problems with age.

The same applies to the necessity for guarding against the loss of effectiveness of the immune and defense systems with age. The most serious risk of a faultering immune system is the formation of an uncontrollable tumor since the defenses are too weak. To a large extent, cancer is actually a normal state in old age, as is arteriosclerosis. Everyone in our civilized world would possibly acquire his or her own cancer if he or she survived long enough, although persons who have an immune system strong enough to survive until the age of 90 or older, appear to have a relative decrease in the incidence of carier.

Cancer in old age in humans, but not in animals, is assumed to be the inevitable result of a life style which no longer suits the species.

The immune weaknesses resulting from old age also explain our increasing susceptibility to infectious disease. In this context, Dr. Fillit of the Mount Sinai Medical Center in New York refers to an age-dependent, AIDS-like immune deficiency. One of the reasons for this immune deficiency in old age is the weakening of the macrophage activity that has already been mentioned several times. The macrophages fail to respond to a mechanism that operates continually in the immune system. It is a fascinating process but not without its dangers.

Put simply, what happens is that a 'lookout' (an antibody) is alarmed so that it can eliminate a second 'lookout' attached to the enemy (antigen). This first 'lookout' attaches itself to both the second 'lookout' and the antigen, and now acts as the mischief-maker by attracting the next 'lookout', thus forming a 'lookout complex' (immune complex). This is a mechanism that forms part of the immune system and operates automatically whether this is good or not. Anything that disturbs us is noticed by the 'lookout' and held on to for destruction.

In more immunological terms, when immune complexes of foreign antigen and the body's own antibodies remain in the system, the result is often the production of a new antibody which is directed against the antibody in the immune complexes, attaches itself to the complexes, attracts the killer enzymes (complement) and so tries to eliminate the undesired immune complexes from the body.

This second antibody, directed against the first antibody, naturally has to possess the correct signature to be able to attach itself, the signature corresponding to the foreign antigen. The first antibody, afterall, is specific for this antigen so that it imitates the foreign antigen. This is known as antigenic mimicry. An anti-antibody of this type is also known as an *idiotype*. This does not imply anything derogatory about its intelligence quotient, the term comes from the Greek and means 'own type'.

Since this idiotype expresses exactly the outer characteristics of the 'bad guy' antigen, the antibodies specifically directed against these characteristics naturally pounce upon the idiotype. Sounds confusing? These are known as anti-anti-antibodies or anti-idiotypes, which again form immune complexes with the idiotypes. Should they not be degraded, and that can happen if the immune system is weakened with age, antibodies can be formed directed against these anti-idiotypes. And so, on and on.

The chain reaction continues ever further and can throw the whole immune system into chaos and paralyze it. Thus, unchecked, uncontrolled complement activation in the wrong places can occur, superfluous fibrin is produced, and immune complex-initiated disorders occur which are identical with the disorders regarded as being typical of old age. There is premature chronic degenerative aging.

The proper destruction and elimination of these pathogenic immune complexes by activated macrophages is essential. According to the European scientists, administration of enzymes is thus a logical way of slowing such age-dependent processes.

Not dying, just ceasing to live

Thus, we alone are responsible and no one else. We are responsible for whether we live healthy lives and consume a natural diet so that our bodies can function optimally as long as possible, whether we reach the limits of our possible life-spans as determined by our genetic makeup.

It is thought that our bodies are so constructed as to be able to live for about 115 years before the genetically determined signal triggers the end. Every death before this time may be regarded as a premature end. Although life expectancy has improved during the past century, traditional myths, stories and the reports of the Old Testament witness that many people in earlier times lived much longer than is usual now.

In the esoteric Indian document, the Upanishad Vedas, the natural life-span of human beings was considered to be 100 years. When the philosopher Arthur Schopenhauer was taught the Indian fables in Weimar by a certain Herr Mayer, the Upanishadic philosophy colored his whole thinking. He also came to the conclusion that we ought to live for one-hundred years.

He wrote, "I am right in my belief. I have observed that only those who have passed the age of 90 years participate in euthanasia, that is die or perhaps do not die but merely cease to live, without disease, without apoplexy, without a shudder, without a death rattle, even sometimes without growing pale, indeed usually sitting after a meal. Earlier deaths result from disease and are premature." Schopenhauer died at the age of 72.

Chapter 18

The future: A world of health?

It sounds like a fairy tale. This vision of a healthy world full of healthy people, free from chronic disease who live to a ripe old age and then end their lives gracefully and easily.

Thousands of highly qualified scientists are working at this moment to realize this world of health. Their successes so far have been splendid and they understand very well, at least in theory, how this long healthy life could be achieved.

Most of the scientists working toward this goal belong to the youngest branch of medicine, immunology. However, you alone can ensure a healthy life with an intact immune system.

The intact immune system depends on an optimal supply of the enzymes required for each process of life. This brings immunologists more and more to a consideration of the questions addressed in this book. By no means has every question been answered, by no means has every experiment been performed. Every problem has not been solved, all the evidence is not yet available and every possibility has not been exhausted.

One aim is to improve and confirm the enzyme therapy that already claims impressive results and finds increasing usage. In the foreseeable future, we can expect to see the perfection of fibrinolysis, to gain control of inflammatory disease, and to be able to prevent, or at least bring to a halt, many cancers and viral diseases as a result of reinforcing the immune system.

Exact control of fibrinolysis by the administration of fibrinolytic enzymes would mean not only that thrombi could be dissolved, but rather it would also allow more reliable prevention of thrombus formation than is possible today. The smallest deposits in the arteries would be removed instantly. The deposition of fats and cholesterol on the artery walls would be prevented to a large extent. The whole vascular system and the tissue interstices would be kept free from the start.

Certainly, the consistent administration of a perfected oral enzyme therapy alone will not be sufficient. A change to a healthy life style is also necessary, from diet to avoidance of nicotine and other toxic substances to adequate exercise, as well as a reduction in exposure to environmental pollutants. It is also a requirement that all these measures be carried out prophylactically, or at least in the early stages of a disorder.

Then, according to the European scientists, "we would certainly come fairly close to our ideal situation: Such important vascular diseases as arteriosclerosis, venous inflammation, thrombosis and embolism, coronary heart disease, circulatory disorders of the brain, lungs, kidneys and liver would be minimized, as would other disorders as well."

They further believe that, "there would no longer be any senile, mentally deranged, disoriented, crippled old people unable to move more than a few steps due to pain. They would see and hear better, remain physically and mentally fit, mobile and active, into their older age, possibly even into the ninth decade.

The complete avoidance of depositions in the vessels and tissues through the use of enzymes would mean a tremendous improvement in the quality of life and an appreciable prolongation of life as well, if indeed confirmed. It would be medical progress unlike any; comparable with the introduction of antibiotics, but superior.

It has already been concluded by some scientists that it is possible to heal contusions and bruises more rapidly, to reduce pain, to promote healing of hematomas and edemas. Other researchers have also concluded that the response of many chronic inflammatory disorders to treatment with enzyme therapy is highly favorable.

Anyone who follows the research on enzyme action closely will realize that we are just at the start. A proper mastery of most chronic inflammatory diseases by the use of improved oral enzyme mixtures is desirable since, in this way, we will be better able to assure the function of the immune system as a whole in the future more than we can now. A proper and assured function of a healthy immune system will make it possible to provide effective treatment of many diseases, and to prevent the many disorders associated with disturbed defense mechanisms.

That will mean relief for millions of suffering people who will be freed from rheumatoid arthritis, most chronic kidney inflammations of immune origin, from chronic progressive inflammation of the liver, the pancreas, the intestinal tract (Crohn's disease and ulcerative colitis), of the lungs, of the arteries (vasculitis), of the nervous tissue (multiple sclerosis) and from many other disorders.

However, the use of enzymes has its limits, what has been destroyed cannot be healed. That would possibly be a task for genetic engineering. Perhaps the further understanding of the genetic code will eventually make it possible to repair defects or even to replace destroyed parts by new growth.

The future of enzyme therapy is closely allied to the complete decipherment of the immune system. We already know a great deal, but every new discovery reveals a little more of its true complicated nature.

This leads us to genetics since we can now say which people are predisposed to which autoimmune disorders on the basis of certain inherited characteristics. The actual outbreak of the autoimmune disease is dependent on further precipitating factors. If diagnosis could be so improved that the programming for predisposition to specific immune diseases could be recognized in time, such people might be helped, according to many scientists, by sufficiently early prophylaxis with enzyme therapy.

Systemic lupus erythematosus (SLE) is but one example for the help that is expected. SLE is a very serious autoimmune disorder that affects the connective tissue of the vessels and whose treatment poses severe problems. A leading theory suggests that it occurs when a genetic predisposition is triggered off by infection with a so-called retrovirus. Immune complexes and antibodies against nucleic acids are then formed, causing severe inflammation in certain regions. The destructive action of complement is triggered which leads to the full SLE disease complex. Many internal organs can be affected in addition to the skin and the vessels.

In animal experiments, the researchers have reported that it has been possible to significantly improve animals suffering from SLE by means of massive doses of enzymes. There are scientific grounds for believing that it will be possible to help human sufferers conquer this severe disease in a similar manner.

The efforts in enzyme research directed at successful treatments of all disorders in which viruses or cancer are implicated are also to be seen in this context. In recent years, the explosive increase of our understanding of immunology makes it evident that one of the principal solutions to the cancer problem will probably not be found in the fields of chemotherapy or radiation therapy, but in the field of immunotherapy.

The future of oral enzyme therapy has already begun. The speed with which this knowledge concerning the scope of enzyme therapy is spreading is truly breathtaking. Nevertheless, the rate at which this knowledge is being applied toward restoring the health of the millions who are suffering unnecessarily is unfortunately surprisingly slow.

This dismays those scientists, physicians, biochemists and pharmacists who are convinced that help is available, but that it is not provided sufficiently on account of prevailing dogma, prejudice, ignorance or lack of courage. In some countries, politically biased laws are difficult to change and, in some instances, take precedence over the promotion of sensible health measures. Evidently, better attention should be paid to preventive measures, and to research of promising treatments of the sick, who could then be helped back to health much better.

This book about enzymes has been written in the hope of advancing the knowledge about enzymes, and hence the day when enzyme therapy will be better accepted and correctly used as a valid therapeutic option in the treatment of a number of disorders where scientists now feel it can be of considerable assistance.

Chapter 19

New developments and current status
of enzyme therapy

Developments and progress in the area of enzyme therapy are occurring at a very rapid pace. Each new publication on this topic carries with it the danger of 'aging'. Those who make use of enzymes are now experiencing a situation similar to that seen with the use of computers as well. Five or even ten years ago, what was considered the ultimate knowledge, today appears somewhat antiquated. This is in part due to the fact that pharmacological research, with its exciting innovations in immunology, is beginning to emphasize the use of biological components which permit the precise operation of the immunological system. "Pharmaceutical Chemistry and Biochemical Pharmacology", an American textbook by Kirk and Othmer, is viewed as a sort of "Bible" to pharmacologists. It states, "in the near future substantial developments in pharmacology and therapeutics can be expected of enzymes."

At least one basic textbook error concerning enzymes which still continues to occupy the minds of some noteworthy professors has been finally corrected and accepted by gastrointestinal absorption experts in America. Namely, the idea that many of the hydrolytic enzymes which are administered to prevent and treat numerous complaints are of such a large molecular size that they cannot be absorbed. Some still think (erroneously according to recent published studies) that these large molecules cannot penetrate the narrow intestinal villi in order to enter the circulatory or lymphatic systems. Therefore, in their view, since they are not absorbed, they cannot be effective throughout the entire organism. Scientific evidence strongly supports the absorption of these molecules, as discussed in the chapter on digestion and in the introduction.

Once again, from the beginning:
Overview of current status of oral enzyme therapy

One other factor blocks the recognition of systemic enzyme therapy in general medicine, which the scientists feel enzymes should already have earned thanks to their reported efficacy. This factor is the skepticism of such physicians who, for instance, have leafed through this short book and, based upon the titles to the chapters, have come to the conclusion that it must be absolute nonsense. You can hear them saying: "Enzymes for multiple sclerosis, rheumatism, inflammations, injuries, cancers, viral infections and complaints of old age. Nonsense!", they will say, "this is one more example of 'hokus pokus', just typical of the many 'wonder drugs' that supposedly heal all illnesses known to man, and yet demonstrate no effects. I can only warn you of them."

Instead of warning, it would perhaps be more suitable to not only read the titles of the chapters, but to read the entire book and pay attention to those chapters concerned with individual illnesses. Many readers only read a few pages in the book concerned with the illnesses in which they are more interested either because of their special occupational interests or because of their own health problems. They are confused and cannot understand the actual nature of enzymes, nor the reason why they function elsewhere in the organism.

They have missed the beginning of the book, the long explanation describing what enzymes actually are. To the easily bored reader, this appears to be only extra effort, excessive talk about things which, as they believe, are 'not easily comprehensible and are nonetheless unimportant'.

It is recommended that the book be read anew and that the entire description of enzymes be absorbed. This is unfortunately a prerequisite for a clear understanding of these unusual therapeutic forms which can be effectively administered for common and important disturbances in health.

It is generally thought that most individual illnesses, regardless of the cause, result in a damaged, interrupted or missing specific immunological step, or a defect of a related component. Thus, if the defect is known, treatment or replacement of the specific factor required is called 'specific therapy'. Enzyme therapy, however, is 'nonspecific' since the same active components are applied for very many illnesses and they are directed to allow the immune defenses to accomplish their jobs by eliminating common obstacles. This does not fit into the concept of many physicians regarding the treatment of certain illnesses with drugs, because they feel more comfortable with specific treatments.

New drugs, new evidence

Those who have never before contemplated the fascinating characteristics of enzymes could of course have difficulties understanding the new uses of enzymes.

Those interested enough in enzymes to read and study this book, can appreciate their importance. Furthermore, if indeed as effective as proposed by the European scientists, and supported by further worldwide scientific research, their use will become more widespread. Likewise, the enzyme mixtures can be constantly improved and further studied in the treatment of other specific medical conditions. Therapeutic effectiveness of enzyme mixtures will help to secure their respected position in medicine.

Thousands of clinical studies in which this new knowledge is being tested and systematically studied are presently taking place throughout the entire world. The Medical Enzyme Research Institute alone has listed more than 125 current studies, investigations and tests in universities, clinics and laboratories. This acquired and applied knowledge naturally leads to constant improvements in therapeutic enzymes and their uses.

The stepping stones in the therapeutic administration of enzyme mixtures have at least been moved closer together with the knowledge gained from numerous studies and publications in scientific journals and books. Consequently, the commercially available enzyme mixtures have been improved twofold. First of all, even more valuable prime materials with a correspondingly higher enzyme yield can be obtained and, secondly, complex pharmaceutical techniques can be used to encapsulate and pack even more highly concentrated enzymes into each tablet.

A result of these changes is the further improved absorption of more activated enzymes in the organism. Even higher potency of the newer, concentrated enzyme mixtures (recognizable through the letter 'N' following the preparation's name) are therefore obtained when the same number of tablets are administered. For instance, 'the *new* anti-inflammatory enzyme mixture' is more potent, tablet for tablet, than the original products. On the other hand, the long-term dose can be reduced if enzymes are taken as prophylaxis or, for instance, if they are to be taken indefinitely for such illnesses as circulatory disturbances.

Even more remarkable is the introduction of a new and more powerful enzyme mixture for systemic enzyme therapy. Namely, this new mixture contains the two enzymes which are most effective for inflammatory illnesses (i.e. bromelain and trypsin) packed into film-coated tablets at double the dose found in the original anti-inflammatory enzyme mixture, and combined with rutin for reducing capillary fragility. The result is an enzymatic preparation especially indicated for acute inflammations, particularly for injuries. This concentrated *rheumatologic enzyme mixture* has a higher concentration of active ingredient in each film-coated tablet and allows reduced dosage. It also has a further advantage. Since the mixture only has three active agents, the cost of the medication is covered by the health insurance companies in some countries, for instance in Germany. Due to its higher concentration and expected higher absorption into the organism, only a few tablets of this mixture are recommended. Studies to this date purport a high degree of effectiveness for acute inflammations, particularly for injuries, as good or superior to the results from the original anti-inflammatory enzyme mixture which has been used for over 30 years.

Swollen ankles and muscle pains

According to the European scientists, the numerous investigations and practical experience gained over the course of years in the field of traumatology, i.e. in wound healing, support the effectiveness of enzyme therapy for acute injuries.

Simple acute injuries are not generally reported and, thus, a precise incidence is lacking from the statistic books. Since they are so commonplace and taken for granted with a sigh, the physician is not even consulted for most of these injuries.

Possibly the best-known example of an acute injury is when we twist an ankle by tripping on a curb or a step so that the ligaments or tendons are slightly overstretched and a swollen ankle results. Likewise, when we bump into the corner of a cupboard, a bruise develops or we suffer from a muscular strain.

Clinical studies were conducted to evaluate individuals who received prophylactic enzyme treatments, or immediate enzyme medical therapy after acute injuries, including professional and competitive athletes who naturally find it important to again take part in sports as soon as possible. As has already been described in this book, the researchers have concluded that when administered before or immediately after an injury, they provide rapid relief by reducing the swelling and pain, and by restoring mobility.

However, does the new concentrated rheumatologic enzyme mixture function equally well? The initial reports of controlled clinical studies have shown that complaints following such injuries as overstretched ligaments and tendons, including sprained ankles, are also improved substantially following treatment with the concentrated rheumatologic enzyme mixtures. Joint swelling and effusion, as well as the limited mobility and pain present when moving the ankle, are all influenced positively.

Reports of clinical studies demonstrated that, without the concentrated rheumatologic enzyme mixtures, injured athletes would be unfit for an average of 6 days and could only begin training after 11 days. Injured athletes treated with the concentrated rheumatologic enzyme mixtures, on the other hand, were only unfit for 4 days and already started training after 8 days. Furthermore, 80% of the patients acknowledged that the concentrated rheumatologic enzyme mixtures demonstrated 'very good' to 'good' results.

This confirmed the findings that traumatologists had already made with the administration of the anti-inflammatory enzyme mixtures. According to them, there seem to be indications that the concentrated rheumatologic enzyme mixtures might even be more effective, and it is also advantageous that 10 or more tablets do not have to be swallowed three times daily for massive-dose therapy since 4 film-coated tablets taken three times a day produce the same effects.

Furthermore, initial studies on the administration of the concentrated rheumatologic enzyme mixtures for athletic injuries have concluded that athletes taking these enzyme tablets prophylactically had fewer severe injuries of the type mentioned than athletes without this protection.

Only slightly more than 10% of injuries due to accidents occur during sports. Thus, the bulk of bruises, strains and sprains, and ordinary contusions which may often cause substantial pain and discomfort, are not sports related. Thus, the most common injuries which cause us trouble, often for weeks, are the result of fully normal, everyday, commonplace situations in approximately 9 of 10 cases.

Theoretically, it would of course be sensible to limit the possible damage. The enzymologists recommend that persons with a history of frequent and severe injuries take the concentrated rheumatologic enzyme mixture tablets after injuries. However, only few individuals would be able to bring themselves to do so. They therefore advise that, as a preventive measure, individuals engaged in high risk activities, like going skiing, mountain climbing, wind surfing, or performing any other athletic activity, consider the use of concentrated rheumatologic enzyme mixtures for prophylaxis during this period.

In their view, this also applies to other physical activities which might result in significant muscular aches. They indicated that enzymes also help to prevent the soreness after extensive physical fitness training. For example, after steadfastly completed jogging, marathon runs or the popular cross-country races, there is quite a chance that one will feel some painful muscles which previously were not even known to exist.

According to the researchers, enzyme preparations like the concentrated rheumatologic enzyme mixtures are more likely to protect one from these muscular pains. They cite the example of weight-lifters who take a large number of the anti-inflammatory enzyme film-coated tablets in order to prevent the risk of injury resulting in muscular soreness.

Risk of injury? Muscular soreness is actually an injury and not merely the result of hyperacidity with lactic acid as was previously assumed. Rather, minor injuries of muscle fibers occur due to the heavy strain placed on particular muscles. Furthermore, there is an inflammatory reaction of the muscle tissue in connection with this and small areas of bleeding into the tissue occur with the formation of small clots and deposition of fibrin. As is the case with every acute inflammation and injury, a great deal of fibrinolytic enzymes of high quality are required for recovery. Our body does not always produce the necessary enzymes in sufficient quantities, sufficiently rapidly or of adequate quality to eliminate all of the fibrin. This is especially true in the elderly where endogenous enzyme fabrication is unfortunately likely to be produced slowly and erroneously.

Dr. Ernst Raas, sports medicine professor at Innsbruck, concerned himself with the prevention of muscle pains in athletes for whom he was in charge (the Austrian alpine ski team as well as others). He also tested this effect on such amateur athletes as the participants of the Karwendel cross-country race which takes place there yearly. The participants are, in part, untrained or improperly trained so that it is no wonder that especially these athletes are often found to demonstrate evidence of muscle damage, such as high creatine kinase levels, following this sporting event. Creatine kinase is an enzyme which plays a role in the accumulation and release of muscular energy, and can therefore be used as a gauge for such muscular damage as seen with sore muscles.

The study included a group of runners who received the enzyme mixtures before the Karwendel run and a control group receiving no enzymes. As expected, the individuals of the control group demonstrated high creatine kinase levels after the run, whereas the values in the runners who had received a prophylactic dose of enzymes remained absolutely normal. These runners also had no typical complaints.

In the professor's opinion, "it therefore appears to be a simple way of protecting oneself from these uncomfortable muscular pains."

Oh dear, my tooth!

Dr. Kurt Vinzenz, university lecturer and senior physician of oral surgery at the New Evangelical Hospital in Vienna, decided to participate for fun in such a race. A sport physician gave him the good advice to take a few enzyme tablets before the race to avoid the muscle pains which would otherwise be almost inevitable. According to Dr. Vinzenz, although he was not very convinced, he took the enzymes anyway and discovered after the race that he, an untrained participant, had no complaints, whereas many well-trained runners complained of severe discomforts.

Shortly thereafter, Dr. Vinzenz participated in a soccer match and in the heat of the moment received a hard kick on the shin. Signs of a hematoma, swelling and pain were seen immediately. This time, the trainer of the soccer club advised him to take a higher dose of the same enzyme mixture. The hematoma and swelling disappeared amazingly quickly and the pain subsided.

Dr. Vinzenz concluded from these experiences that if the severity of the pathological condition was limited by the prophylactic administration of enzymes and these conditions could be alleviated more readily through prompt administration of these enzymes, it must also function in the same way for the intentional injuries to which he, as an oral surgeon, subjected his patients daily with the extraction of wisdom teeth or some other oral surgical procedure. Afterall, as already mentioned in this book, every operation is an intentional bodily injury.

In order to test his theory, Dr. Vinzenz performed a randomized, double-blind study on 80 patients who had to undergo oral surgical procedures. About half of the patients received the actual enzyme mixture, whereas the remaining patients received a placebo which could not be differentiated visually from the effective tablets. Neither the physician nor the patient knew whether a particular patient was receiving the enzymes or the placebo.

According to Dr. Vinzenz, "the key to the code was disclosed after the study had been completed and it was established that patients treated with the enzymes generally tolerated the drug 'very well'. Nearly 90% of them also evaluated the drug efficacy as being 'very good' or 'good'. All laboratory values that could be indicative of inflammatory processes revealed more favorable levels in the patients treated with enzymes. The improvement in the general state of health, the regression of swallowing difficulties and the reduction of lymph node swelling were also significant for these patients."

Further studies and daily practical experience lead Dr. Vinzenz to "the realization that, 2 to 3 days after removal of the wisdom tooth, the patients could already eat without problems if they had taken high doses of the enzyme mixtures 48 hours before surgery. Without this enzymatic protection, the complaints required 10 to 12 days to improve."

He also felt that the danger of bacterial infection of the wound by organisms living in the oral region was also reduced in the patients who took the enzymes, a danger which can have potentially serious effects, especially for certain cardiac cases where the release of bacteria can lead to endocarditis.

Dr. Vinzenz believes that, "the fear that such enzymes could increase the risk of bleeding, or that bleeding from the operative site could possibly be hard to control, are exaggerated." He emphasized that a good oral surgeon has no problem with bleeding wounds.

Dr. Vinzenz determined such parameters of bleeding as the so-called prothrombin time and the bleeding time. The prophylactic enzymes were given at appropriate doses before any operation was performed and no significant changes in bleeding parameters were observed.

More substantial than possible bleeding from damaged vessels are 'seeping hemorrhages'. These entail the much more dangerous extravasation of proteinaceous plasma substances or cellular fragments, from the serum and tissue into the interstitial spaces. Dr. Vinzenz pointed out that, "the risk of actual seeping of these proteinaceous and cellular fragments is actually reduced through the administration of the enzyme mixture. The surgeon may therefore have to treat small vessels which tend to bleed following prophylactic enzyme treatment, but can still administer additional enzymes during surgery." Like him, other scientists also feel that there will be a lower risk with respect to the dangers of 'seeping hemorrhage' thanks to these enzymes.

Alleviation of rheumatic pain

Toothaches are generally short-lived since the causes are known and something can be done about them. However, how is it for the millions of people who suffer from rheumatism day in and day out?

Some of the causes of the countless illnesses related to rheumatism are beginning to be discovered, but that is little consolation for the patients who want relief from their often excruciating pains here and now. There is no wonder drug which can cure all so-called 'rheumatic' illnesses. Even the potent enzyme mixtures are not a wonder drug of this kind. However, they are purported to provide as much or more assistance than the other traditional drugs most frequently prescribed, without the risks of side effects found with these conventional drugs.

Scientists feel that, "the administration of enzyme mixtures has proven to be highly effective and reliable in repeated studies, especially for patient groups afflicted with chronic arthritis." In addition, the efficacy has also been tested in other soft tissue illnesses, also classified within the vague rubric of 'rheumatic' illnesses.

The so-called ankylosing spondylitis (Marie-Strumpell arthritis or Bekhterev's arthritis), a chronic and very painful inflammation of the intervertebral joints of the lower back, is also a member of this category of rheumatic illnesses which can, in the course of time, lead to a curvature and then to a stiffening of the spine. Little is known about the precise etiology of this inflammation, although it is generally thought to represent a variant of rheumatoid arthritis. The therapy is correspondingly difficult.

Dr. Klaus-Michael Goebel, a professor at the Rheumatological Clinic in Bad Endbach, Germany, reported that nearly half of the patients suffering from this chronic inflammatory illness, Bekhterev's arthritis, demonstrated large-molecular immune complexes flowing in their bloodstreams. Based on the literature, reports describing the rheumatologic enzyme mixtures as having a positive influence on inflammatory processes and as being able to decompose circulating, pathogenic immune complexes, Professor Goebel decided to perform a prospective, long-term, randomized, double-blind study utilizing the conventional anti-inflammatory agents in comparison with the new rheumatologic enzyme mixtures. Half of the patients suffering from Bekhterev's arthritis received the rheumatologic enzyme mixtures, whereas the other half received the commonly prescribed, nonsteroidal anti-inflammatory agent indomethacin or a placebo.

According to him, the patients treated with indomethacin were seen to have a substantially more rapid reduction in pain during the initial four months of observation than those receiving the rheumatologic enzyme mixtures. However, after the first four months, a significant change then occurred, indomethacin became less effective and the pains once again became more severe. At this point, the rheumatologic enzyme mixtures, on the other hand, became increasingly more effective against pain than indomethacin and the reduction in pain lasted for a longer period even after therapy was discontinued.

Whatever parameters Professor Goebel examined, it could clearly be seen that the rheumatologic enzyme mixtures were initially slower to take effect than indomethacin, although in the long term it functioned more effectively and more prolonged. In the course of time, 16 patients of the rheumatologic enzyme mixture group revealed improvement in the mobility of the lumbar spine. It achieved a continuous reduction in the circulating immune complexes after four weeks, whereas the concentration of circulating immune complexes in the indomethacin group increased to such an extent that the general condition of these patients deteriorated.

Professor Goebel therefore advised his colleagues to prescribe the rheumatologic enzyme mixtures together with indomethacin during the first few weeks in order to motivate the impatient and suffering patients to continue with the drug administration because of the rapid alleviation of pain. He recommended that the rheumatologic enzyme mixtures be given alone thereafter in order to avoid the threatening negative effects of indomethacin which often occur with long-term administration. The same principle applies to the use of prednisone or systemic corticosteroids for acute inflammatory arthritis.

The term 'rheumatism' does not only include rheumatic complaints of the joints or bones, but unfortunately also a large number of illnesses in which the muscles and tissue are affected with these rheumatic inflammations.

Rheumatism of the soft tissue represents a similar problem for the medical sciences as the arthroses and chronic inflammatory, arthritic illnesses of the joints. Laboratory examinations scarcely provide clarity; the symptoms are often ambiguous. The treatment of the various complaints which occur under the collective term 'rheumatism of the soft tissues' is highly unsatisfactory. In the long run, the treatment is usually burdened with adverse effects which can occasionally become even more severe than the actual rheumatic symptoms.

The predominant symptom for the patients is pain. Naturally, the swelling of the affected soft-tissue structures, the limited mobility, the muscle stiffness and the hardening of the muscles are also uncomfortable. However, the pain bothers the patients most since it is felt with movement or even at rest, and is sometimes present constantly. It makes life hardly bearable day or night, and remains the dominant therapeutic problem. Unfortunately, treatment of rheumatism of the soft tissues remains largely symptomatic, and no specific treatments directed against the causes or its cure are available.

Dr. Klaus Uffelmann, a physician from Gemünden, Bavaria, in cooperation with 24 other private practitioners, performed a clinical study involving 424 patients suffering from rheumatism of the soft tissues. The patients were treated with enzyme mixtures. Following treatment with an enzyme mixture, the researchers recognized substantial improvements in the complaints of patients suffering from myositis (inflammation of the muscles) and tenosynovitis (inflammation of the tendons).

All 424 patients had previously received treatment with the usual drugs without any noticeable effects. Half of the patients received the rheumatologic enzyme mixtures and the other half a placebo which looked identical. Reportedly, after eight weeks, the patients treated with the rheumatologic enzyme mixtures revealed significant improvements in active and passive movement, morning onset pains and nightly pains. The pain on pressure, the limitation in mobility, the soft-tissue swelling and the hardening of the muscles were considerably reduced.

According to Dr. Uffelmann, the rheumatologic enzyme mixtures were tolerated excellently. They concluded that, regarding overall response, effectiveness and tolerance, the enzymes were considered to be superior to the commonly prescribed nonsteroidal anti-inflammatory agents. Furthermore, as was already observed in the therapy of the other rheumatic illnesses, the positive effect of the rheumatologic enzyme mixtures persisted even after the drug was discontinued.

Help for women

It is a good sign when an increasing number of specialists in various fields decide to treat with a drug which is claimed to have an effect on multiple and diverse ailments, although it has a debatable reputation because it is nonspecific. One could say that, for these reasons, the drug raises 'questions'. However, in spite of this, an increasing number of physicians are now using enzyme mixtures. For example, gynecologists in Europe are now using enzyme mixtures to treat certain diseases in women which could not be treated suitably with the usual drug schemes. They are using enzyme mixtures, either alone or in combination with other traditional treatments.

Pelvic inflammatory disease

One of these specialists is Professor Dittmar, senior physician of the gynecological-obstetrics department of the District Hospital in Starnberg, Germany. He has administered the enzyme mixtures successfully for many years in the treatment of such women's disorders as adnexal illnesses (inflammation of the fallopian tubes and/or the ovary), mastopathy (benign alterations in the female breast) and malignant tumors. He has also treated endometriosis, a difficult condition associated with painful menses and pelvic discomfort due to benign deposits of cells originating in the uterine lining which grow beyond the uterus and get inflamed during the hormonal cycles.

In the scientific papers published by Professor Dittmar on this topic, he describes, for example, the traditional treatment of acute and especially of subacute and chronic adnexal illnesses as often being difficult and lengthy. The patients suffer from pain, are less able to handle day-to-day activities and are generally less active. There are scars, adhesions, degenerative symptoms in the affected ovaries, an uncomfortable vaginal flora (discharge), disturbances in the menstrual cycle and, last but not least, the danger of sterility. The drugs which are available and usually administered can only be given with great reservations and for short time periods since their side effects are problematic for women of child-bearing age.

Due to these reservations, Professor Dittmar looked for an alternative which could be accepted from a medical standpoint and was also reasonable for the patients. He reported that he had found this alternative in the anti-inflammatory enzyme mixtures.

This assumption gained support in a comparative, clinical, double-blind study performed by Professor Dittmar on 56 patients with adnexitis. Half received the anti-inflammatory enzyme mixtures and the other half received placebos. On the average, there was complete improvement in the anti-inflammatory enzyme mixture group and no change in those receiving placebo. The evaluation of clinical effectiveness of the anti-inflammatory enzyme mixtures was reported as being very good.

This form of treatment has meanwhile become standard therapy in his department. "The patient receives the anti-inflammatory enzyme mixtures immediately as an acute therapy and, in many cases, also to avoid such late symptoms as sterility and chronic adhesive inflammations." Enzymes during the acute phase are considered adjuvant treatment. Therapy with the absolutely mandatory antibiotics cannot be replaced by this drug.

Benign cysts of the breast

Positive results found in studies with the enzymatic treatment of cystic disease of the breast (mastopathy) at other clinics have supported the findings of Professor Dittmar.

Chronic cystic disease of the breast (mastopathy) in the form of benign changes in the tissue of the breast is reported to affect about half of all women of child-bearing age. The patients have such complaints as dragging or stabbing pains in the region of the axilla, as well as tenderness on pressure, and pain on tension and swelling. The complaints are often more severe before the menstrual period.

Clearly effective treatment of mastopathy does not exist. A number of physicians, such as Dr. Scheef from the Janker Clinic in Bonn, Germany, used enzyme therapy for this condition. He reported relief of the complaints and thereby minimized the understandable fear of possible breast cancer.

In order to affirm these findings, Professor Dittmar performed a double-blind study on 96 patients suffering from mastopathy. Forty-eight patients were treated with the enzyme mixtures and 48 with a placebo. After six weeks, the complaints of the women in the placebo group remained unchanged, whereas those from the enzyme group had improved appreciably. Although the number and size of benign cysts in the placebo group had not changed, there was a reduction in the size of cysts in the enzyme group.

An approach to breast cancer

The greatest fear of every woman with tissue changes in the breast is naturally the fear of having breast cancer. Improved operative methods with excellent cosmetic results after breast reconstruction, as well as the advances in chemotherapy and in some cases radiation, has helped to remove much of this terrible fear of breast cancer. Whenever possible, patients should be reassured. When one considers all age groups, the possibility that a woman will die of other causes is higher. Overall, death from cardiovascular disease is more than 12 times as high as that of dying from breast cancer. More women die from inflammation of the lungs, flu, asthma or other illnesses of the respiratory tract than from breast cancer.

However, this does not alter the fact that breast cancer continues to be the most frequent carcinoma in women and represents a serious threat. In the treatment of a cancerous illness, everything should be done to ensure the patient a life with minimal complaints for as long as possible and with as little cosmetic impairments as possible.

The operative removal of the tumor is the most important measure. In addition, dependent on the growth of the tumor, radiation and chemotherapy may be considered. Previously, this therapeutic scheme did not provide entirely satisfactory results. Not only were numerous patients cosmetically and psychologically altered by radical mastectomies, but cancer 'nests' were left behind or may have been accidentally 'seeded' in the operative region in many surgical procedures, with the subsequent risk of dissemination.

This major risk has been reduced through effective surgical sealing of the afferent and efferent vessels in the operative region. Afterall, the death from a tumor is not what is generally to be feared, rather death resulting from cancer metastases which have been spread throughout the body via blood and lymphatic vessels.

A second risk involves the immune system which has been weakened by radiation and chemotherapy. It is important for every cancer patient who has had a tumor removed surgically that the body's immune system be assisted and not weakened. Afterall, this immune system must come to terms with the cancer cells remaining in the organism, must detect them, track them down, hold them tight and destroy them. The 'immune security' must function.

The Viennese oncologic surgeon, Dr. Ottokar von Rokitansky has been concerned for years with the control of these two risks in the treatment of breast cancer. He has gained a great deal of experience in this regard, and has reported results which, according to him, are superior to those usually found.

According to Dr. von Rokitansky, these results are dependent on the meticulous care with which the surgical technique is performed, a procedure in which only the tumor and those additional tissues which are absolutely necessary are excised. He also reported that it depends on the care with which the body's own immune system is supported.

This care already begins one to two weeks before the operation. Dr. von Rokitansky "injects the oncologic enzyme mixtures into and around the tumor daily, and occasionally more than once a day, in a dose which he feels is suitable for combating the cancer." In addition, "he also administers these enzyme mixtures in the form of oral tablets or via enemas."

In cases of more advanced or dangerous tumors, and if the breast cancer patient is not pregnant, Dr. von Rokitansky also treats with high doses of vitamin A. He administers 200,000 IU daily.

Following the operation, the patient is again treated with the enzyme mixture in tablet form, daily for one week each month, continued for a number of years. He feels that the use of this post-operative treatment gives the cancer patients a better chance to live longer and with a higher quality of life, a belief which has already been described in the chapter dealing with cancer.

The results from Dr. von Rokitansky are quite impressive. He has reported on the results with 305 patients who underwent surgery for breast cancer and were followed-up for more than 10 years.

Accordingly, he reported that the ten-year survival rate (five years of survival from cancer is also referred to as 'the five-year cure') for patients with Stage I breast cancer was approximately 85%. Generally, patients with the more severe Stage II tumors demonstrate lymph nodes with metastatic involvement. In Dr. Rokitansky's study, the ten-year survival rate for patients with more severe Stage II cancer was reported as being more than 75%. These results compare favorably with other studies of Stage I and II breast cancer, but direct comparison with equivalent patients treated with standard adjuvant chemotherapy both with and without enzymes should be performed. Anyone familiar with the comparative survival rates in other studies can appreciate how encouraging these results are.

Because of its great importance for the further well-being of patients who have undergone surgery, lymphedema of the axillary region, a typical and rightfully feared sequel following breast operations, will again be considered here shortly. It is not the same thing as metastatic involvement of the lymphatic ducts and lymph nodes. Rather, it represents a progressive swelling due to the damaged lymphatic vessels. This develops in certain breast cancer patients in connection with tissue damage during the surgery and with extravasation of plasma protein into the tissue interstices. This liquid is then transported away insufficiently because of interrupted lymphatic vessels which were damaged as well, and congestion or edema subsequently results. A vicious cycle of mutually increasing disturbances begins whose most evident result is the swelling of the afflicted axillary region as far as the clavicle and extends to the entire upper arm. A swelling which can become as hard as a board and occasionally is so unshapely that one speaks of elephantiasis. The edema causes discomfort and continuously limits the mobility of the arm, ever increasingly. A superimposed danger is that this lymphedema can progress to yet another different type of cancer of the damaged lymphatic and blood vessels known as lymphangiosarcoma or Stewart-Treves Syndrome.

This is not the place to introduce all the sensible measures for treating such surgically-dependent lymphedemas which extend from dietary tips, to gymnastics, to manual lymphatic drainage. Rather, it should once again be repeated here that, according to experienced European oncologists, this dreaded consequence of a breast operation can usually be avoided. Dr. Wolfgang Scheef, from the Janker Clinic in Bonn has reported that lymphedemas only appeared within two years in 4.5% of the breast cancer patients who had undergone surgery while under prophylactic treatment with an anti-inflammatory enzyme mixture, whereas, in other studies, up to 26% of these patients who did not receive this enzyme protection suffered from lymphedema.

When medicine harms us

Sometimes there is no alternative, we must undergo medical therapy which is expected to help us, but which unfortunately also produces some damage. As we have seen, this is true of every operation and, even more so, of the often immunosuppressive radiation and chemotherapy.

In every oncologic clinic, one is aware of the damages to which the cancer patient is subjected. They are accepted as being unavoidable. Naturally, every responsible physician attempts to keep the exposure to radiation and chemotherapy as low as possible by improvements in instrumentation and limitation of this treatment to the absolutely mandatory minimum.

Dr. Michael Schedler in Homburg, Germany, is a physician who is principally responsible for the follow-up treatment of cancer patients at the university clinic. He was responsible for the management of patients with very advanced conditions, some of whom had been treated with radiation therapy and chemotherapy. The question arose as to whether systemic enzyme therapy might be able to help in these severe cases. The researcher concluded that the enzyme treatment provided considerable improvement in the general state of health and strengthened the body's resistance. This improvement, he felt, resulted in a reduction of damages caused by the radiation and chemotherapy and a subsequent reduction in the risk of metastasis.

As an additional therapy, he also administered the oncologic enzyme mixtures and extremely high doses of vitamin A to cancer patients with very advanced illnesses before and after radiation or chemotherapy. According to him, after evaluation of 109 of these cases, the patients were seen to have substantially fewer side effects to the usual radiation and chemotherapy than patients who were not treated using this therapeutic scheme.

In his study, he included other types of cancer seen at the university oncologic clinic. One result of this study was especially noteworthy. Bleomycin is one of the most important chemotherapeutic agents in the treatment of tumors in the region of the ears, nose and throat used for arresting cell division. However, the excellent efficacy of bleomycin cannot be fully exploited since the lungs tend to be damaged severely as a side effect. The most effective dose which is thus far recognized as being the upper limit that can be recommended has up to a 15% chance that a very serious and, at times, potentially fatal respiratory disturbance might develop.

According to Dr. Schedler, this lung damage complication has not even occurred once since he administered the oncologic enzyme mixtures concurrently to every treatment with bleomycin at the University Clinic in Hamburg. Dr. Schedler then increased the bleomycin dose gradually until it was doubled and has so far not been forced to discontinue therapy because of this fearful respiratory damage.

A study by the university lecturer Dr. Friedrich Beaufort from the University Radiological Clinic in Graz, Austria, provided information concerning the limitation of damage in cancer patients treated with radiation therapy. The radiation often destroys the healthy tissue surrounding the tumor to differing degrees. For example, in bladder tumors thus treated, local inflammation, skin irritation, even inflammation of the mucosa of the bladder and cystitis can result from the massive necrosis which occurs. Radiation therapy always leaves a 'battlefield' of cellular debris and extravasation of fluids from the blood vessels and tissues at the site of exposure.

In a study on 57 patients with cancer in the region of the abdomen, Dr. Beaufort examined the capabilities of an oncologic enzyme mixture for clearing up this 'battlefield' and influencing the inflammation in the affected region. Although patients treated with enzymes revealed side effects to radiation therapy similar to those also seen in patients who received no enzymes, there were significant differences. According to him, these complaints lasted an average of less than 14 days in the enzyme treated patients. In contrast, they lasted nearly four weeks in the unprotected patients. The repair of the damage brought about by the radiation therapy was achieved nearly twice as rapidly after enzyme administration.

The European researchers point out that this chemotherapy sparing effect is, so to speak, an encore to the favorable influence in reducing the metastatic potential of the tumor, and an encore to the reinforcement of the body's immune system in the cancer patients who were treated with enzymes. Likewise, they point out that, "another significant contribution is the replacement of a drug with serious side effects with an equally effective enzyme mixture which is as good, but free from side effects."

When the immune system harms us or becomes depressed

The Enzyme Research Institute contends that this therapeutic enzyme effect has recently been documented and justified scientifically, offering valid alternatives for the treatment of two more illnesses. Namely, the use of the rheumatologic enzyme mixtures as an alternative to the use of oral gold therapy in chronic inflammatory arthritis and use of the enzyme mixtures as an alternative to acyclovir, a drug which has so far been recognized as being most effective, in shingles, i.e. herpes zoster. In both cases, the researchers reported that the enzymes offered comparable positive effects, nearly without the negative side effects which commonly occur with the other drugs.

The first results of a randomized, controlled, double-blind, multicenter study under the direction of Dr. Michael-W. Kleine from Planegg, Germany were concluded comparing oral enzymes and acyclovir. A total of 96 zoster patients were studied. The alleviation of pain, the early healing of vesicles and the reduction of crusting were basically equal for both drugs in the same period of time; there was no difference seen here between enzyme and acyclovir therapy. However, while enzyme treatment was as good as acyclovir, it was superior as far as being free from side effects. The possible side effects of acyclovir, although admittedly low, are well-known to every physician. Lately, renal disturbances have been reported with acyclovir.

More importantly, in Dr. Kleine's study, the enzyme group developed no post-herpetic neuralgia, while the acyclovir had no apparent effect in reducing the dreaded neuralgia.

Other researchers, as mentioned in the section on the enzymes' activity against viruses, have reported that this type of enzyme offers at least an inhibitory effect on the HIV illnesses leading to AIDS.

Can AIDS be treated?

It is understandable if physicians react with skepticism as soon as a new concept for the treatment of HIV illnesses is reported. Too much hope has been shattered, too many reports of success have at least proven to be premature and too many adventurers have attempted to make a quick fortune from the troubles of the afflicted.

To once again justify the submitted material on the treatment of HIV positive individuals with enzymes, we quote from a special publication by Dr. Hans Jäger, from Munich, Germany, one of the most experienced European physicians in the treatment of AIDS, and chairman of the Committee for Immunodeficiency.

Anyone who has read this book and the explanation of circulating immune complexes will surely understand what Dr. Jäger has reported. A few of the specialized terms will therefore be translated into general layman's English.

According to Dr. Jäger, "There are increasing indications that autoimmune processes play a role in the destruction of the immune system and in the development of the HIV illness. Among other things, various autoantibodies and an elevated level of circulating immune complexes (CIC) are found. The CIC level in patients afflicted with HIV is related to the course of the illness. It could play a role in the development of the immunodeficiency via complement-transmitted cellular destruction. Dr. Jäger and associates postulate that hydrolytic enzymes are able to mobilize tissue-fixed immune complexes and to eliminate circulating immune complexes directly or by way of macrophage activation. Results of the first pilot study on patients with early stages of the illness (WR 1–5) revealed a good tolerance of the enzyme therapy, an improvement in body weight and in the general activity of the patient. Although the T helper cells were unchanged, there was a reduction in the amount of clinical symptoms typical for HIV."

"Again, a controlled examination following a therapy-free interval of one month revealed a deterioration of most of these parameters. However, individual patients reported subjective improvements when the enzyme therapy was restarted. The enzyme therapy was tolerated well, only a few reversible side effects occurred, including disturbances in the gastrointestinal tract."

"A further pilot study in Frankfurt with 15 patients in Stage LAC/ARC has been running now for over two years." In the last report, "five of these patients were practically free of symptoms with enzyme therapy alone, whereas the other 10 patients required additional antiviral therapy."

"More extensive, multicenter studies have already begun in New York City (HIV infected patients with more than 500 helper cells) and Berlin (HIV infected patients with classical symptoms). A monotherapy with hydrolytic enzymes cannot be recommended for clinically advanced stages or for patients with substantial reduction of immunological functions. Again, enzymes should be considered adjuvant therapy. Here, the enzymes are given in combination with antiviral and other agents, and the treatment should be considered supportive therapy."

With this in mind, the enzyme researchers have concluded that enzyme therapy has a capability of mobilizing cell-bound immune complexes, and degrading those complexes which are circulating in the vessels. They also postulated other mechanisms, thus offering a treatment alternative for the pre-AIDS stages, before the outbreak of the actual AIDS disease.

We must wait for the results of the ongoing studies, and other studies planned, in order to see where and to what extent the enzyme therapy can be used to actually help control the suffering of this threatening AIDS epidemic. The scientific authorities have no longer shut themselves off from this possibility and are now working on converting this theory into practice, in America as well.

New insights into how enzymes work

A most fascinating and important role of enzyme therapy has been recently reported. The researchers reported a direct action of hydrolytic enzyme mixtures on very important biological substances known as adhesion molecules. These can be best described as 'hooks, tentacles or suckers' which are apparently pressed out from every cell and are used to connect or anchor these cells to other cells, membranes or tissues. In this way, a large junction of equivalent cells can build a stable unit. The organs, for example, are held together in this way and do not disintegrate into a cellular porridge.

Cancer cells are able to form imitations of the suckers of certain organs and can therefore adhere to the cells of these organs. The enzymes can apparently differentiate between the true suckers and the imitations by the cancer cells, and can then break away the adhesion molecules, thus making these proteinaceous counterfeits less of a problem.

These are fascinating ideas for every scientist which are being investigated to the utmost and supported by substantial research grants at the present.

It can therefore be acknowledged that even this "Enzyme" book cannot portray the final state of knowledge. Nothing is more stable than change.

We conclude this book by repeating our belief that enzymes represent a highly promising modality of medical treatment. They represent 'the medicines of the future' and their use is likely to increase as we learn more about the immunopathology of diseases and conduct more clinical and scientific studies utilizing them.

Glossary of Medical Terms

Anemia	A general term describing conditions where there is a reduction in the content of pigment in the red blood cells and a general reduction in the number of these cells.
Anticoagulants	Drugs inhibiting or delaying the clotting of blood.
Arteriosclerosis	Hardening of the arteries, the most frequent arterial disorder. Formation as a result of degeneration of the arterial blood vessels with loss of elasticity (hardening) of the vessel walls.
Bekhterev's disease	Ankylosing spondylitis or Marie Strümpell disease; chronic inflammatory disease of the spinal column, the intervertebral disks and joints adjacent to the spinal column through the involvement of immune complexes.
Clones	Multiplication of genetically uniform descendants of a mother cell.
Crohn's disease	Chronic inflammation of the small intestine as a result, at least in part, of lymph obstruction by immune complexes; usually progressive in stages.
Double-blind study	Method of testing the efficacy of a medicinal preparation where neither the subject being tested nor the physician or assistant performing the investigation knows whether the preparation or a placebo (inert substance disguised as the preparation) is being administered.

Embolism	Sudden obstruction of a blood vessel by a blood clot which has moved there from another site.
Exudate	Fluid that can escape from the affected vessels during inflammation.
Fibrinolysis	The enzymatic dissolution of fibrin, the substance formed to produce blood clots.
Hemodialysis	Blood washing (artificial kidneys); the artificial removal of metabolic wastes and toxins from the bloodstream as a replacement for faulty kidney function.
Hemophilia	A disease of the blood; genetically inherited defect leading to inhibition of blood clotting.
Immune complex	A combination of foreign antigen with the antibodies formed by the body to combat these substances. If these are not degraded, pathogenic reactions may result.
Immunosuppressive	Drug for the artificial suppression of the body's natural defenses.
Infuse, to	Administration of liquids into the organism, usually via the veins.
Lupus erythematosus	A sun-sensitive disease producing inflammation of the vessels as a result of undegraded immune complexes which leads primarily to changes in the skin, but also to changes in the joints and internal organs.
Lymphedema	Collection of tissue fluids exuded by chronically affected and, hence, congested and inflamed lymph vessels.

Lymphapheresis	Artificial drainage via the main lymph duct of the body (thoracic duct), enabling withdrawal of lymphocytes.
Multicenter study	A study where the same investigation is performed simultaneously in several medical practices or hospitals.
Mutation	A finite change in the structure or effect of one or more hereditary factors which persists.
Oral	By mouth, here in the sense of the route of administration.
Pancreatitis	Acute or chronic inflammation of the pancreas.
Phlebitis	Inflammation of venous vessels with varying participation of the vessel wall.
Photosynthesis	Production of energy-rich compounds by conversion of light energy into chemical energy.
Plasmapheresis	Separation of the liquid plasma from the solid fraction or cellular components of the blood after removal. The cells are then returned to the circulation in foreign plasma or salt solution.
Pulmonary fibrosis	Pathological growth of connective tissue in the lungs leading to a restricted function.
Rebound effect	Excess production and excretion of certain endogenous (from within the body) substances (e.g., hormones) after the inhibition of these substances has ended.
SLE	Systemic lupus erythematosus (see Lupus erythematosus).

Systemic	A systemic effect is one exhibited by an organ system or the entire body.
Thrombocyte activation	Thrombocytic platelet activation is triggered by a factor secreted by the activated cell for this purpose. This causes the thrombocytes to secrete certain proteins and to aggregate to a certain extent.
Thrombocyte aggregation	Aggregation of thrombocytes which takes place in two phases. This plays an important role in blood clotting and thrombus formation.
Thrombosis	Partial or complete obstruction of a blood vessel by the presence of a blood clot (thrombus).
Toxoplasmosis	Illness brought about by parasites which cause congenital disorders, usually transmitted to people from animals.
Traumatology	The science concerned with the cause, prevention and treatment of injuries.
Ulcerative colitis	Chronic inflammation of the mucosa of the large intestine with ulcerative destruction of the intestinal wall.
Vasculitis	General term for vessel inflammations of all types.

References

Adams, D. O. et al.: Phagocytic cells: Cytotoxic activities of macrophages. In: Gallin J. I., Goldstein I. M., Snyderman R. (Eds.): Inflammation – basic principles and clinical correlates. Raven Press, New York, 1989.

Adibi, S. A.; Mercer, D. W.: Protein digestion in human intestine as reflected in luminal, mucosal, and plasma amino acid concentration after meals. J. Clin. Invest. 52: 1586 – 1594 (1973).

Amborse, A. M.; De Eds, F.: Effects of rutin on permeability of cutaneous capillaries. Pharmacol. Exp. Ther. 90: 359 (1989).

Ambrus, J. L. et al.: Absorption of exogenous and endogenous proteolytic enzymes. Clin. Pharmacol. Ther. 8: 362 (1967).

Aschner, M. S.; Sheppard, H. W.: AIDS as immune system activation: a model for pathogenesis. Clin. Exp. Immunol. 73: 165 – 167 (1988).

Avakian, S.: Further studies on the absorption of chymotrypsin. Clin. Pharmacol. Ther. 5: 712 (1964).

Baintner, K.: Intestinal absorption of macromolecules and immune transmission from mother to young. CRC, Boca Raton, FL (1986).

Baltimore, D.; Lodish, H.; Darnell, J.: Molecular cell biology. Scientific American Books, New York (1990).

Barrett, A. J.; Starkey, P. M.: The interaction of α-2m with proteinases. Biochem. J. 133: 709 (1973).

Barrett, A. J.: Proteinases in mammalian cells and tissues. Elsevier, North Holland Biomedical Press, 1977.

Barsom, S.; Sasse-Rollenhagen, K.; Bettermann, A.: Successful prostatitis treatment with hydrolytic enzymes. Experience Therapy (Erfahrungsheilkunde) 31: 2 (1982).

Barsom, S.; Sasse-Rollenhagen, K.; Bettermann, A.: Treatment of cystitis and pyelocystitis with hydrolytic enzymes. Acta Medica Empirica 32: 125 (1983).

Bartsch, W.: Treatment of zoster with proteolytic enzymes. The Informed Physician 2: 424 – 429 (1974).

Baumgartner, G.; Baumgartner, M.: Results of a pilot study with enzymes in addition to cytostatic therapy for malignant diseases. Viennese Clinical Weekly (Wiener Klin. Wochenschrift) 97: 148 (1985).

Baumhackl, U.; Fordermair, S.: Enzyme therapy in multiple sclerosis. A preliminary report on a multicenter study. General Medicine (Allgemeinmedizin) 19 (4): 169 – 172 (1990).

Baumüller, M.: XXIV FMS World Congress of Sport Medicine. Symposium on Enzyme Therapy in Sports Injuries. May 29, 1990, p 9. Elsevier Science Publishers, Amsterdam (1990).

Beard, J.: Enzyme therapy of cancer. In: Wolf, M. (Hrsg.) Maudrich-Verlag, Vienna (1971).

Beaufort, F.: Reduction of side effects of radiation therapy with hydrolytic enzymes. Therapeutikon 10: 577 – 580 (1990).

Bender, B. S. et al.: Role of the mononuclear phagocyte system in the immunopathogenesis of human immunodeficiency virus infection and the acquired immunodeficiency syndrome. Rev. Infect. Dis. 10: 1142 – 1154.

Bjarnason, I.; Peters, T. J.: Helping the mucosa make sense of macromolecules. Gut 28: 1057 – 1061 (1987).

Blazar, B. A. et al.: Circulating immune complexes and chemotherapy response in patients with head and neck cancer. Head Neck 11: 431 – 436 (1989).

Blonstein, J. L.: Oral enzyme tablets in the treatment of boxing injuries. Practitioner 198: 547 (1967).

Bockman, D. E. et al.: The role of epithelial cells in gut-associated immune reactivity. Ann. NY Acad. Sci. 409: 129 – 143.

Bohe, M. et al.: Fate of intravenously injected trypsin in dog with special reference to the existence of an enteropancreatic circulation. Digestion 29: 159 (1984).

Bongrand, P.: Physical basis of cell-cell adhesion. CRC Press, Boca Raton (1988).

Boyer, P. D. et al.: Editors: Fruton, S.: The enzymes, Vol. 4, Academic Press, New York (1960).

Brambell, F. W. R.: The transmission of immunity from mother to young and the catabolism of immunoglobulins. Lancet 11: 7473 – 7475 (1966).

Brambell, F. W. R.: The transmission of passive immunity from mother to young. Frontiers of Biology, Vol. 18, North-Holland, Amsterdam (1970).

Buch, S. P. et al.: A prospective study of circulating immune complexes in patients with breast cancer. Int. J. Cancer 41: 364 – 370 (1988).

Buch, S. P. et al.: Human lung cancer – a comparative study of the levels of circulating immune complexes in pulmonary blood draining the tumor area and peripheral venous blood. Int. J. Cancer 42: 837 – 840 (1989).

Buch, S. P. et al.: Primary lung cancer. A controlled study of preoperative and postoperative levels of circulating immune complexes. Cancer 61: 2033 – 2041 (1988).

Bugis, A. et al.: Inhibition of lymphokine-activated killer cell generation by blocking factors in sera of patients with head and neck cancer. Cancer Immunol. Immunother. 31: 176 – 181 (1990).

Carini, C. et al.: Complement activation is associated with the presence of specific HIV-anti HIV immune complexes in patients with ARC of LAS. Second J. Immunol. 30: 347 – 353 (1989).

Chain, E.; Duthie, E. S.: Identity of hyalurinodase and spreading factor. J. Exper. Pathol. 21: 324 (1940).

Colony, P. C.; Neutra, M. R.: Macromolecular transport in the fetal rat intestine. Gastroenterology 89: 294 – 306 (1985).

Dasgupta, M. K. et al.: Circulating immune complexes in multiple sclerosis: relation with disease activity. Neurology 32: 1000 – 1004 (1982).

Daugharty, H. et al.: Immunoglobulin bound to platelets as immune complexes or specific antibody in specimens from AIDS and immune thrombocytopenic purpura. Diagn. Immunol. 3: 205 – 214 (1985).

Debanne, M. T.; Bell, R.; Dolovich, J.: Uptake of proteinase-α-macroglobulin complexes by macrophages. Biochem. Biophys. Acta 411: 295 (1975).

DeSmet, P. A.; Pegt, G. W.; Meyboom, A. H.: Acute circulatory shock following administration of the non regular enzyme preparation Wobe-Mugos®. Nederlands Tijschrift voor Geneeskunde 135: 2341 – 2344 (1991).

Desser, L.; Rehberger, A.: Induction of tumor necrosis factor in human peripheral-blood mononuclear cells by proteolytic enzymes. Oncology 47: 474 (1990).

DeVita, V. T. J. et al.: Developmental therapeutics and the acquired immunodeficiency syndrome. Ann. Intern. Med. 106 (4): 568 – 581 (1987).

DeVita, V. T.; Hellmann, S.; Rosenberg, S. A.: Cancer – principles & practice of oncology. J. B. Lippincott Company, Philadelphie, Toronto (1982).

Dittmar, F. W.: Enzyme therapy in gynecology. General Medicine (Allgemeinmedizin) 19 (4): 158 – 159 (1990)

Dittmar, F. W.: Enzyme therapy in inflammatory pelvic disease. The Medical World (Die Medizinische Welt) 37: 562 – 565 (1986).

Dobryszycka, W. et al.: Acute phase reactants and circulating immune complexes in patients with ovarian carcinoma. Archivum Immunolgiae et Therapieae Experimentalis 39: 41 – 50 (1991).

Dorrer, R.: Treatment of malignant tumors with Wobe-Mugos® preparations. Experience Therapy (Erfahrungsheilkunde) XIV 8: 373 – 377 (1965).

Dulbecco, R.: Progress in cancer research: Proceedings of the 4th international conference on progress in cancer research. San Remo, Italy (1989).

314   *Enzymes – The Fountain of Life*

Dulbecco, R.; Ginsberg, H. S.: Virology. J. B. Lippincott Company, Philadelphia, Toronto (1988).

Dunkel, R.: Therapy investigations with proteolytic enzymes in camel pox. Veterinary Review (Tierärztliche Umschau) 11: 580 (1973).

Ekerot, L. K.; Ohlsson, K.; Necking, L.: Elimination of protease-inhibitor complexes from the arthritic joint. Int. J. Tissue Reac. VII: 391 (1985).

Emele, J. F.; Shanaman, J.; Winbury, M. M.: The analgesic-anti-inflammatory activity of papain. Arch. Int. Pharmacyn. Ther. 159: 126 (1966).

Esparza, I. et al.: Inhibition of macrophage tumoricidal activity by immune complexes and altered erythrocytes. J. Immunol. 131: 2117 – 2121 (1983).

Euler, H. H. et al.: Precipitable immune complexes in healthy homosexual men. AIDS and the related LAS. Clin. Exp. Immunol. 59: 267 – 275 (1985).

Fauci, A. S.: The human immunodeficiency virus: Infectitity and mechanism of pathogenesis. Science 239: 617 – 622 (1988).

Fiasse, R. et al.: Circulating immune complexes and disease activity in Crohn's Disease. Gut 19: 611 – 617 (1978).

Felix, E.: Oral activity of pharmaceuticals used in venous diseases. Therapy Week (Therapiewoche) 11: 1083 (1986).

Fillit, H. M. et al.: Antivascular antibodies in the sera of patients with senile dementia of the Alzheimer's type. J. Gerontol. 42 (2): 180 – 184 (1987).

Fruton, S.: Cathepsins A-C in The Enzymes. Editors: Boyer, P. D. et al., Vol. 4: 233 – 241, Academic Press, New York (1960).

Fukodome, J. S.; Yoshikawa, M.: Opioid peptides derived from wheat gluten: Their isolation and characterization. FEBS Lett. 296: 107 – 111 (1992).

Gaggi, R.; Biagi, G. L.: Mutagenicity study of Wobenzym®. Report from the Institue of Pharmacology at the University of Bologna (1985) (Document entry)

Gaggi, R.; Biagi G. L.: Pharmacotoxicologic Study of Wobenzym®. Report from the Institue of Pharmacology at the University of Bologna (1985).

Ganrot, P. O.: Studies on serum protease inhibitors with special reference to α-2 macroglobulin. Acta. Univ. Lund. Sect. II 2: 1 (1967).

Garnder, M. L. G.: Intestinal assimilation of intact peptides and proteins from diet – a neglected field? Biol. Rev. 59: 289 – 331 (1984).

Gaschler, A.: The parenteral ferment therapy of malignant tumors and chronic inflammation. Pharma Laboratory Gaschler, Lindau, Lake Constance.

Gebert, G.: Enteral resorption of intact protein molecules. General Medicine (Allgemeinmedizin) 19 (4): 125 – 131 (1990).

Gifford, G. E.: Tumor necrosis factor. Microbiol. Sci. 5: 104 – 107 (1988).

Goebel, K. M.: Enzyme therapy in ankylosing spondylitis. In: Medical Enzyme Research Society. Systemic Enzyme Therapy, 17th Meeting, Vienna (1991).

Goldberg, D. M.: Enzymes as agents for the treatment of disease. Clin. Chimi. Acta 206: 45 – 76 (1992).

Götze, H.; Rothman, S. S.: Amylase transport across ileal epithelium in vitro. Gastroenterol. Clin. Biol. 3: 298 (1979).

Götze, H.; Rothman, S. S.: Enteropancreatic circulation of digestive enzymes. A conversation mechanism. Nature 257: 607 (1975).

Gruskay, F. L.; Cooke, R. E.: The gastrointestinal absorption of unaltered protein in normal infants and in infants recovering from diarrhea. Pediatrics 16: 763 – 769 (1955).

Guggenbichler, J. P.: Influence of hydrolytic enzymes in thrombi formation and thrombolysis. Medical World (Med. Welt) 39: 227 (1988).

Hall, D. A. et al.: The effect of enzyme therapy on plasma lipid levels in the elderly. Atherosclerosis 43: 209 (1982).

Hand, R.: Alternative therapies used by patients with AIDS. N. Engl. J. Med. 320 (10): 672 – 673 (1989).

Hechter, O.; Salomon, S.: Spreading phenomenon and inflammation. Nature 162: 701 (1948).

Hechter, O.: Mechanism of spreading factor action. Ann. N Y Acad. Sci. 52: 1028 (1959).

Heinrich, H. C. et al.: Enteropancreatic circulation of trypsin in man. Clinical Weekly (Klin. Wochenschr.) 57: 1295 (1979).

Heinrich, H. C.; Gabbe, E. E.; Brüggemann, J.; Icagic, F.: Classen, M.: Enteropancreatic circulation of trypsin in man. Clinical Weekly (Klin. Wochenschr.) 57: 1295 (1979).

Heinz, H. P.; Loos, M.: Activation of the first component of complement, C1: Comparison of the effects of 16 different enzymes on serum C1. Immunobiology 165: 175 – 185 (1983).

Hemmings, W. A.: Transport of large breakdown products of dietary protein through the gut wall. Gut 19: 715 – 723 (1978).

Heumann, D.; Vischer, T. L.: Immunomodulation by α-2 macroglobulin and α-2 macroglobulin-proteinase complexes: The effect of the human T-lymphocyte response. Eur. J. Immunol. 18: 755 – 760 (1988).

Hiss, W. F.: Enzymes in sport medicine and traumatology. Journal for Natural Therapy Methods (Zeitschrift für Naturheilmethoden) Volume 2: 1 (1979).

Hodgson, H. J. F. et al.: Immune complexes in ulcerative colitis and Crohn's disease. Clin. Exp. Immunol. 29: 187 – 196 (1977).

Hörger, I.; Moro, V.; van Schaik, W.: Circulating immune complexes in patients with polyarthritis. Natural and Hollistic Medicine (Natur- und Ganzheitsmedizin) 1: 117 – 122 (1988).

Howell, E.: Enzyme nutrition. Avery Publishing Group, Inc., Wayne, NJ 1985.

Inderst, R.: Enzyme therapy in vascular diseases. General Medicine (Allgemeinmedizin) 19 (4): 154 – 157 (1990).

Inderst, R.: Systemic enzyme therapy. Journal of Pharmacy 52 (1992).

Isaaksson, J. I.; Ihse, I.: Pain reduction by oral pancreatic enzyme preparation in chronic pancreatitis. Dig. Dis. Sci. 28: 97 – 102 (1983).

Iseman, L. D.; Rothman, S. S.: The transport of protein through the basolateral membrane of pancreatic acinar cell. Physiologist 18: 259 (1975).

Jäger, H. et al.: Hydrolytic enzymes as biological response modifiers (BRM) in HIV-infection. In: San Marino Conferences – Highlights in Medical Virology, Immunology and Oncology, Volume 1: 44, San Marino, Pergamon Press, Oxford, New York, Tokyo, Toronto (1988).

Jäger, H.: Hydrolytic enzymes in the treatment of HIV disease. General Medicine (Allgemeinmedizin) 19 (4): 160 – 164 (1990).

Johnson, K. J.; Peter, A. W.: Newer concepts in the pathogenesis of immune complex induced tissue injury. Lab. Invest. 3: 218 (1982).

Jutila, M. A. et al.: Low dose chymotrypsin treatment inhibits neutrophil migration into sites of inflammation in vivo. Effects on adhesion protein expression and function. Cell. Immunol. 132: 201 – 214 (1991).

Kameke, E. v.: Enzyme cascades in plasma – how can they be utilized therapeutically? Experience Therapy (Erfahrungsheilkunde).

Kameke, E. v.: Inflammation and its treatment with hydrolytic enzymes and rutin. Forum of the General Practitioner (Forum des Praktischen- und Allgemeinarztes) 9 (1981).

Kim, J. -P.; Hah, W.-S.; Kim, S.-J.: Effects on rosette forming T-lymphocyte level in immunochemotherapy using Picibanil and Wobe-Mugos® in gastric cancer patiens. J. Corean. Surg. Cos. 23 (1981).

Kiprov, D. D. et al.: The role of apharesis procedures as an immunoregulatory therapy in patients with AIDS related conditions. J. Cell Biochem. [Suppl.] 8: 22 (1984).

Kirk-Othmer: Pharmaceutical Chemistry & Biochemical Pharmacology.

Klein, G.; Pollmann, G.; Kullich, W.: Clinical experience with enzyme therapy in patients with rheumatoid arthritis in comparison with gold. General Medicine (Allgemeinmedizin) 19 (4): 144 – 147 (1990).

Klein, G.; Schwann, H.; Kullich, W.: Enzyme therapy in chronic polyarthritis. Natural and Hollistic Medicine (Natur- und Ganzheitsmedizin) 1: 112 – 116 (1988).

Kleine, M.-W.; Vogler, W.: Systemic enzyme therapy. Introduction and overview. General Medicine (Allgemeinmedizin)19 (4): 119 – 124 (1990).

Kleine, M.-W.; Pabst, H.: Action of an oral enzyme therapy in experimentally induced hematomas. Forum of the General Practitioner (Forum des Praktischen- und Allgemeinarztes) 27: 42 (1988).

Kleine, M.-W.; Pabst, H.: The effects of an oral enzyme treatment on experimentally induced hematomas. Forum of the General Practitioner (Forum des Praktischen- und Allgemeinarztes) Volume 2: 27 (1988).

Kleine, M.-W.: Treatment of herpes zoster with proteolytic enzymes. Therapy Week (Therapiewoche) 37: 1108 – 1112 (1987).

Krc, I. et al.: Crohn's disease, serum immunodepressive factors and circulating immune complexes. Sieroter Boll Milan 59: 619 – 624 (1980).

Kunze, R. et al.: Humoral Immunomodulatory Capacity of Proteases in Immune complex Decomposition and Formation. First International Symposium on Combination Therapies, Washington, D. C. (1991).

Laffaioli, R. V. et al.: Prognostic significance of circulating immune complexes in a long-term follow up of breast cancer patients. Oncology 45: 337 – 343 (1988).

LaMarre, J. et al.: Cytokine binding and clearance properties of proteinase-activated α-2 macroglobulin. Laboratory Investigation 65: 3 – 14 (1991).

Larrick, J. W.: Therapeutic Enzymes for Cancer, Special Presentation, Biologic Response Modifiers Symposium, Tulsa, Oklahoma, October 1992.

Layer, P. et al.: Fate of pancreatic enzymes during small intestinal aboral transit in humans. Am. J. Physiol. Gastrointest. Liver Physiol. 251: 475 (1986).

Liebow, C.; Rothman S. S.: Enteropancreatic circulation of digestive enzymes. Science 189: 472 (1975).

Lightfoote, M. M. et al.: Analysis of immune complex components isolated from serum of AIDS patients. Fed. Proc. 43: 1921 (1984).

Lightfoote, M. M. et al.: Circulating IgA immune complexes in AIDS. Immunol. Invest. 14: 341 – 345 (1985).

Lindner, A.; Förster O.: Report on the influence of Wobenzym® in different rat foot – pad edemas. Scientific Monograph (1976).

Maehder, K.: Enzyme treatment in diseases of the veins. Medical Practice (Die Arztpraxis) Volume 2 (1978).

Mahr, H.: Enzyme treatment of inflammatory venous diseases, of deep vein thrombosis and of post-thrombotic syndrome. Experience Therapy (Erfahrungsheilkunde) 32: 117 – 121 (1983).

Matthews, D. M.: Protein absorption – then and now. Gastroenterology 73: 1267 – 1279 (1977).

Matthews, D. M.: Protein absorption. Wiley-Liss, New York (1992).

McDoucal, J. S. et al.: Immune complexes in the acquired immunodeficiency syndrome (AIDS). J. Clin. Immunol. 5: 130 – 138 (1985).

McHugh, T. M. et al.: Relation of circulating levels of HIV antigen, antibody to p24, and HIV-containing immune complexes in HIV-infected patients. J. Infect. Dis. 158: 1088 – 1091 (1988).

Menzel, E. J.; Runge, S.: Enzymes as immunomodulators. General Medicine (Allgemeinmedizin) 19 (4): 140 – 143 (1990).

Menzel, E. J.; Werk, W.: Study on the absorption of Wobenzym®. Report from the immunological Institute of the University of Vienna and the Medical Enzyme Research Institute, Munich (1978).

Messerschmidt, G. L. et al.: Protein A immune adsorption in the treatment of malignant disease. J. Clin. Oncol. 6: 203 – 212 (1988).

Miehlke, K.: Enzyme therapy in rheumatoid arthritis. Natural and Hollistic Medicine (Natur- und Ganzheitsmedizin) 1: 108 (1988).

Miyata, K. et al.: Interaction between serratia protease and human plasma α-2 macroglobulin. J. Appl. Biochem. 2: (1980).

Miyata, K. et al.: Intestinal absorption of serratia protease. J. Biochem. 89: 1231 (1981).

Mörl, H.: Management of the post-thrombotic syndrome with a mixture of enzymes. Therapy Week (Therapiewoche) 36: 2443 – 2446 (1986).

Morrow, W. J. W. et al.: Circulating immune complexes in patients with immune deficiency syndrome containing the AIDS-associated retrovirus. Clin. Immunol. Immunopathol. 40: 515 – 524 (1986).

Mycek, M. J.: Cathepsins A-E. Methods Enzymol. 19: 285 – 315 (1970).

Nagayama, H. et al.: Clinical application of plant protease (Kimotab) in surgical field. Arch. Jpn. Chic. 35: 395 (1966).

Nakahara, M. et al.: Intestinal plasminogen proactivator and activator after oral administration of proteolytic enzymes. Pharmaceutical Research (Arznei-mittelforschung) 17 (1967).

Nakazawa, M. et al.: Proteolytic enzyme treatment reduces glomerular immune deposits and proteinuria in passive Heymann nephritis. J. Exp. Med. 164: 1973 – 1987 (1987).

Netti, C.; Bandi, G. L.; Pecile, A.: Anti-inflammatory action of proteolytic enzymes of animal, vegetable or bacterial origin administered orally compared with that of known antiphlogistic compounds. Il Farmaco Ed. Pr. 27: 453 (1972).

Neuhofer, C. H. et al.: Pathogenic immune complexes in multiple sclerosis: Their elimination by hydrolytic enzymes – a therapeutic approach. International Multiple Sclerosis Conference, Rome, Sept 14 – 17, Monduzzi Editore S. p. A., Bologna (1988).

Neuhofer, Ch.: Enzyme therapy in multiple sclerosis. Hufeland Journal 2: 47 – 50 (1986).

Nielsen, L. R. et al.: Analysis of the decreased NK (natural killer) activity in lung cancer patients, using whole blood versus separated mononuclear cells. J. Clin. Lab. Immunol. 29 (2): 71 – 77 (1989).

Oldham, R. K.: Principles of cancer biotherapy. Raven Press, New York, 1991.

Ostade, X. V. et al.: Human TNF mutants with selective activity on the p55 receptor. Nature 361: 266 – 269 (1993).

Ow, D. W. et al.: Heavy metal tolerance in the fission yeast requires an ATP-binding cassette-type vacuolar membrane transporter. Embo Journal 11: 3491 – 3499 (1992).

Ow, D. W.; Schneider, M.; Howell, S.H.: The vivo pattern of firefly luciferase expression in transgenic plants. Plant Molecular Biology 14: 935 – 947 (1990).

Owgang, C. et al.: Feedback regulation of pancreatic enzyme secretion: Suppression of cholecystokinin release by trypsin. J. Clin. Invest. 77: 2042 – 2047 (1988).

Papp, M. et al.: Absorption of pancreatic lipase from the duodenum into lymphatics. Experienta 33: 1191 (1977).

Paroli, E.: Opioid peptides from food. World Rev. Nutr. Diet 55: 58 – 97 (1988).

Petersen, C. M. et al.: Bioactive human recombinant tumor necrosis factor-alpha: an unstable dimer? Eur. J. Immunol. 19: 1887 – 1894 (1989).

Price, N. C.; Stevens, L.: Fundamentals of Enzymology. Second Edition, Oxford University Press, 1989.

Purcell; Barnhardt: Cathepsin D enhances the proteolysis of prothrombin to thrombin and thus plays an important role in blood clotting. Biochem. Biophys. Acta 78: 800 (1963).

Raas, E.: Institution of enzyme therapy in traumatology. In: MEF (editor): Systemic Enzyme Therapy 4th Meeting (March 1988). Medipharma relations, Munich 17 – 18 (1988).

Rahn, H.-D.; Kilic, M.: The action of hydrolytic enzymes in traumatology. Results after two prospective randomized double blind studies. General Physician (Allgemeinarzt) 19 (4): 183 – 187 (1990).

Rahn, H.-D.: Hydrolytic enzymes as peri-operative anti edematous therapy in meniscectomy and fracture surgery. Presented at the FIMS World Congress of Sports Medicine, May 27 – June 1 (1990).

Ransberger, K. et al.: Natural medicine therapy of AIDS with enzyme preparations. Forum of the General Practitioner (Forum des Praktischen- und Allgemeinarztes) 4: 27 (1988).

Ransberger, K.: Enzyme therapy of cancer. Therapeutics (Die Heilkunst) 102: 22 – 34 (1989).

Rayn, R. E.: A double blind clinical evaluation in the treatment of acute sinusitis. Headache 7: 13 (1967).

Reinbold, H.; Maehder, K.: The biological alternative in the treatment of inflammatory rheumatic diseases. Journal for General Medicine (Zeitschr. f. Allgemeinmedizin) 57: 2397 – 2402 (1981).

Rokitansky, O.: The surgical treatment of carcinoma of the breast with adjuvant enzyme therapy. Dr. med. 1 – 2: 16 – 24 (1980).

Rosenberg, Z. F.; Fauci, A. S.: Immunopathogenic mechanisms of HIV-infection. Clin. Immunol. Immunopathol. 50: 149 – 156 (1989).

Rosner, L. J.; Ross, S.: Multiple Sclerosis: New hope and practical advice for people with MS and their families. Prentice Hall Press, New York (1987)

Roy, S.; Wainberg, M. A.: Role of mononuclear phagocyte system in the development of acquired immunodeficiency syndrome (AIDS). J. Leukoc. Biol. 43: 91 – 97 (1988).

Runowicz, C. D. et al.: Immune complexes in ovarian carcinoma. Gynecol. Oncol. 32: 350 – 353 (1989).

Ruyssen, R.; Lauwers, A.: Pharmaceutical enzymes. E. Story-Scientia PB. A., Gent, 1978.

Samter, M. et al.: Immunological diseases. Little, Brown & Co., Boston, 1988.

Sanella, L. S.: Effect of testicular extract on distribution and absorption of subcutaneous saline solution. Yale J. Biol. Med. 12: 433 (1940).

Schedler, M. et al.: Adjuvant therapy with hydrolytic enzymes in oncology – hopeful effort to avoid Bleomycinum induced pneumotoxicity? J. Cancer Res. Clin. Oncol. 116: 1 (1990).

Scheef, W.; Pischnamazadeh, M.: Proteolytic enzymes as a simple and safe method for the prevention of lymphedema after mastectomy. Med. World (Med. Welt) 35: 1032 – 1033 (1984).

Scheef, W.: Benign changes of the female breast. Therapy Week (Therapiewoche) 35: 5909 – 5912 (1985).

Scheef, W.: Enzymtherapie. Text book of natural medicine procedures. Bd. II, S. 95 – 103 (Hrgs. K.-Ch. Schimmer), Hippokrates-Verlag 1987.

Schleicher, P.: Immune complexes and autoaggression. Natural and Hollistic Medicine (Natur- und Ganzheitsmedizin) 1: 103 – 107 (1988).

Seifert, J. et al.: Quantitative analysis about the absorption of trypsin, chymotrypsin, amylase, papain and pancreatin in the G.I. tract after oral administration. General Physician (Allgemeinarzt) 19 (4): 132 – 137 (1990).

Seifert, J.; Ganser, R.; Brendel, W.: Absorption of proteolytic enzymes of plant origin from the G.I. tract into the blood and lymph of adult rats. German Journal of Gastroenterology (Z. Gastroenterol.) 17: 1 (1979).

Seifert, J.; Siebrecht, P. et al.: Amylase absorption and transport via blood and lymph after oral administration. Digest Biol. Sci. 41: 1593 (1986).

Seifert J. et al.: Qualitative analysis about the absorption of trypsin, chymotrypsin, amylase, papain and pancreatin from the G.I. tract after oral adminstration. General Physician (Allgemeinarzt) 19: 132 (1990).

Slaff, J. I. et al.: Protease-specific suppression of pancreatic exocrine secretion. Gastroenterology 87: 44 – 52 (1984).

Smith, R. A.; Baglioni, C.: The active form of tumor necrosis factor is a trimer. J. Biol. Chem. 262 (15): 6951 – 6954 (1987).

Starkey, P. M.; Barrett, J.: Chymotrypsin like enzyme. Catalytic and immunological properties. Biochem. J. 155: 273 (1976).

Starkey, P. M. et al.: Cathepsin G. Isolation from the human spleen. Biochem. J. 155: 255 (1976).

Stauder, G.; Pollinger, W.; Fruth, C.: Systemic enzyme therapy. A review of the new clinical studies. General Medicine 19 (4): 188 – 191 (1990).

Stauder, G.; Streichhan, P.; Steffen, C.: Enzyme therapy – a complete description. Natural and Hollistic Medicine (Natur- und Ganzheitsmedizin) 1: 68 – 89 (1988).

Stauder, G. et al.: Adjuvant therapy of HIV infections with hydrolytic enzymes: Course of neopterin, CD4 T-cells, immune complexes (IC), and clinical efficacy. 8th International Workshop of Biochemical and Clinical Aspects of Peridines. St. Christoph (Tyrol), Febr. 11 – 18 (1989).

Stauder, G. et al.: Randomized prospective trial of adjuvant use of hydrolytic enzymes in abdominal cancer patients given radiotherapy. German Journal for Oncology 23: 7 (1991).

Stauder, G. et al.: The use of hydrolytic enzymes as adjuvant therapy in AIDS/ARC/LAS patients. Biomed. Pharmacother. 42: 31 – 34 (1988).

Steffen, C.; Menzel, J.: Enzyme consumption from immune complexes. Journal for Rheumatology (Zeitschrift f. Rheumatologie) 42: 249 – 255 (1989).

Steffen, C.; Menzel, J.: Basic investigation on enzyme therapy in immune complexes. Vienna Clinical Weekly (Wien. klin. Wochenschrift) 97: 376 (1985).

Steffen, C.; Menzel, J.: In-vivo destruction of immune complexes in the kidneys after the administration of oral enzymes. Vienna Clinical Weekly (Wien. klin. Wochenschrift) 15: 99 (1987).

Steffen, C.; Menzel, J.: Basic investigation of enzymatic treatment of immune complex disease. Vienna Clinical Weekly (Wien. klin. Wochenschrift) 97: 3 (1985).

Steffen, C.; Menzel, J.; Smolen, J.: Intestinal absorption of an enzyme mixture (Wobenzym®) labeled with 3H. Acta Medica Austriaca 6: 13 (1979).

Stojanow, G.: Metastasis overview, metastasis prophylaxis and tumor treatment with enzymes from the standpoint of the gynecologist. Austrian Journal for Research and Treatment of Cancer 5: 25 (1970).

Streichhan, P.; Pollinger, W.; van Schaik, W.; Vogler, W.: G.I. tract absorption of oral enzymes, in particular Wobenzym®. Journal for General Medicine (Zeitschr. f. Allgemeinmedizin) 65: 716 – 722 (1989).

Temin, H. M.; Baltimore, D.: RNA-directed DNA synthesis and RNA tumor viruses. Virus Research 17: 129 – 186 (1972).

Theofilopoulos, A. N.: Evaluation and clinical significance of circulating immune complexes. Prog. Clin. Immunol. 4: 63 – 106 (1980).

Tilz, G. P.; Becker, H.: Antigen antibody complexes – physiology and pathology. General Medicine (Allgemeinmedizin) 19 (4): 138 – 139 (1990).

Travis, J.; Salvesen, S.: Human plasma proteinase inhibitors. Ann. Rev. Biochem. 52: 655 (1983).

TW Magazin: Advances in the battle of cancer. Therapy Week (Therapiewoche) 38 (1988).

TW Magazin: Systemic enzyme therapy – Present status and advances. Therapy Week (Therapiewoche) 37 (1987).

Uffelmann, K.; Vogler, W.; Fruth, C.: The use of proteolytic enzymes in extra-articular rheumatism. General Medicine (Allgemeinmedizin) 19 (4): 151 (1990).

Vellini, M. et al.: Possible involvement of eicosanoids in the pharmacological action of bromelain. Pharmaceutical Research (Arzneimittelforschung) 36: 110 – 112 (1986).

Vincenz, K.: Action and tolerance of Wobenzym® in the treatment of edema in surgical dentistry. Conclusions of a randomized double-blind study. Maxillofacial surgical clinic. University of Vienna. AK Vienna1989.

Vogler, W.: Enzyme therapy of soft tissue rheumatism. Natural and Hollistic Medicine (Natur- und Ganzheitsmedizin) 1: 123 – 125 (1988).

Walford, R. L. et al.: Selective inhibition of elastolytic and proteolytic properties of elastase. Arch. Biochem. Biophys. 98: 191 – 196 (1962).

Werk, W.; Hörger, I.: The immune profile of rheumatoid arthritis patients before and after enzyme therapy (including a discussion of the mechanism of effectiveness) LAB. J. Res. Lab. Med. VII: 273 (1980).

Weston, et al.: Cathepsin D involved in the catabolism of cartilage and connective tissue. Nature 222: 285 (1969).

White, J. R.: The clinical use and side effects of insulin therapy. Pharm/Alert 1 (1) 1 – 5 (February 1993). Adapted from Clinics in Pediatric Medicine and Surgery: Pharmacology 9 (2) 239 – 255 (April 1992).

Wigzell, H.: Immunopathogenesis of HIV-infection. J. AIDS 1: 559 – 565 (1988).

Wolf, M.; Ransberger, K.: Enzyme therapy. Maudrich-Verlag, Vienna 1970.

Wörschhauser, S.: Conservative therapy in sports injuries. Enzyme preparations for treatment and prophylaxis. General Medicine (Allgemeinmedizin) 19 (4): 173 (1990).

Wrba, H.: Treatment of cancer with proteolytic enzymes. In: Wrba H. (editior): Combined Tumor Therapy pp. 131 – 145, Hippokrates-Verlag, Stuttgart 1990.

Yamada, K. M.: Fibronectins – adhesive glycoproteins. Nature 275: 179 – 184 (1987).

Index

E

F

G

H